Mastering Health

Stretch fascia, oxygenate, strengthen and enlighten.

Book 1: The Active Stretch

By Dr. Eric Pastrmac DC, ND

Photographs by Michael Markovic
Design and Editing by Cathy Wilson

Table of Contents

The secret formula to healing your back.

Introduction

Oxygenate, Stretch, Strengthen, Meditate and Heal.

I would like to introduce you to a system of deep diaphragm breathing and twist or torque stretching, utilizing your own strength to do so. In this sense, our system is sort of a Yoga, since Yoga means union of the spirit and the body. In this sense, our DDB 15/10 is type of an extreme yoga. *Spiritus* in Latin means breath. Deep diaphragmatic breath is intense breathing; we are practicing intense spirit entering the body, taking our energy to stretch to an optimum level.

You are about to embark on a 21-day rehab program that will change your life forever—that is, if you participate. Like anything else, what you put into it, you will get back.

This started out as a self-help book for managing spinal pain, but these principles of diaphragmatic breathing, relaxing the mind, and freeing nerve roots, apply to all healing. Your brain is actually within your body. It actually controls and communicates with everything. When I say everything, I mean everything. The way your brain gets within your body is between the bones of your spine via the nerve roots.

1

Over one billion people worldwide suffer day in and day out with back pain, neck pain, shoulder pain, and headaches. According to The American Academy of Pain Management, in the US alone, we currently spend between $560-635 billion annually for loss of work, doctors, physical therapy, drugs, and devices to resolve our pain. If you are one of these people, there are several important facts about all of this suffering you should know.

The human spine was never intended for man to walk on his hind legs, and misalignment of the spine, according to Hippocrates, the father of medicine, is the root cause of all disease. If man were to get down on all fours, the spine would fall perfectly into place. But when standing, the vertebrae above shift posterior. This shifting is dramatically exaggerated especially in the lower back when in sitting position and should slide back in proper position when standing. However this is not always the case. When bones remain in a misaligned position, discs can't hydrate properly. This is one of the main reasons our spines degenerate, a condition named osteoarthritis. Our vertebrae are constantly going through a great balancing act to keep our head erect and eyes parallel to the ground. This is called the ocular reflex balance. If particular bones are fixated, "subluxated," they would cause other bones to shift. Shifting would have to also accommodate the ocular reflex. All this bone shifting causes absolute havoc on the nervous system, organ functions, and cortisol levels. This in turn causes stress, compromises longevity, and long-term, and may cause irreparable internal damage. It is only through pain that our body can alert us that something is not right. However, pain gone unaddressed will immobilize and degenerate the body regardless of age. These degenerative, osteoarthritic, changes can be seen on the X-Rays of the spine.

What can be done to prevent all of this? Unfortunately, not much, unless you want to walk around on all fours with the family dog. There is good news, though: your spine can be healed. As a doctor of chiropractic, I would start by strongly recommending you seek out the expertise of a knowledgeable, well-trained chiropractor, one that really takes the time evaluate each individual's needs, through consultation and X-Rays. The X-Ray evaluation process is invaluable since it allows the doctor to look at the spine and skull that house the brain and spinal cord, the essence of life, so he or she can figure out the root causal issues that will actually correct the problem and diminish pain.

So how exactly does all of this healing business work? Your brain is inside your body. Think about it for a second. Our brains are actually not just in our head but also extend from the head down the spinal cord, and then via nerve roots extend into the body, dividing, branching, encompassing every organ and communicating with 100 trillion cells in your body.

Nerve roots are extensions of the nerve webs, and nerve webs are extensions of the spinal cord, and the spinal cord is an extension of the brain. Simply put, the brain creates the signals, information, or think of it as thought, that heals the body. Without the brain, nothing in the body would work at all! The following pages will reveal a self-help method showing you how to open the spine, allowing a better flow of data through these neuronal webs from the brain to the body's cells, or simply put, give the body self-healing information.

The Origin of DDB 15/10

The deep diaphragmatic breath held for 15 seconds, then
released for 10 seconds, with increased intensity.

The system I am about to share with you was born
out of personal necessity. A few years ago, I started to
experience incapacitating shoulder pain created by
years of neglect. This escalated into immobility and
failure to take my joints to their normal range of
motion. Despite my routine chiropractic adjustments,
the repetitive stress of daily life was not allowing my
shoulder to heal. Quietly, stiffness, entropy, atrophy,
and degeneration creep up on you, unnoticed.
Something more needed to be done. Then it clicked! I
needed to develop my own rehab program.

Trying to figure out the perfect routine, I remembered
the ancient breathing system revealed to me by the
late Master Tung, a Chinese medicine man and
modern day healer. I met Master Tung at a health
expo. We became friends after he realigned my knee
that had a full ACL tear. Surgery never ensued. He
applied deep diaphragmatic breathing to help realign
the muscles around the joint. I learned a lot from
him. Part of his muscle realignment technique was a
deep diaphragmatic breath held until the vein on
your forehead seemed ready to burst. I adapted this
theory of breath with my own fascia twist stretch, and

I was on to something big! This new system fixed my shoulder pain, rehabilitated my lower back injury, and literally saved my neck. And so, to the benefit of hundreds of my patients, Deep Diaphragmatic Breath, 15 in, 10 out, was born, or as I have coined it, DDB 15/10.

Everything goes through birth, growth, atrophy, entropy, and change of state into a new order. This holds true for all forms of life on the planet. In fact, stars, and even galaxies are not exempt from this cycle. We are all aging, in our perceived reality, and sooner or later, the energy of life begins to diminish. Men's testosterone levels are at their peak in their 20's and begin to drop thereafter. Likewise, women's progesterone and estrogen levels are in perfect balance in our teens through our twenties and then begin to diminish. And so similarly, our connective tissue, fascia, muscles, and joints are in optimum form in youth and tend to stiffen over time. The cycle of life continues, and although this program was originally developed for the stiff and aging, it applies as a conditioning program for all ages, sexes, and abilities.

The DDB 15/10 program is designed to oxygenate and stretch the fascia and muscles. It also increases energy and vitality, corrects posture, and strengthens body and mind. DDB 15/10 serves as a fantastic "recovery day" workout for all muscles and connective tissue. It can also be used as a pre-workout for elite athletes who need to prime the body by eliminating stiffness and gaining mental clarity before serious competition. Done with proper focus and intensity, it is a workout in itself. It was designed to bring back the youthful vitality and flexibility that we all crave.

Note on Breath

Find peace in your body and mind as you become more aware of turning points of inhalation and exhalation of your deep breath.

Breathing with your diaphragmatic oxygenates and relaxes.

We often forget how to breathe. As babies, our diaphragm works great. We start out as belly breathers and all is good. Time goes by and we forget. We forget the joys, freedom, wonder, thrill and excitement of seeing or learning something new. We get caught up. A program begins to form and we either catch it, or as in most cases, it catches us. This programming runs deep, stemming back to government, churches, parents, ancestors, or society. We forget our innocence; we forget the love we came from, the holy creation. We become separate from the whole, essence, or being. When this happens, we begin to feel very alone in this world and we begin to have fears. As A.E. Housman, nineteenth century poet, put it, "Alone and afraid in the world I never made." Fear perpetuates stress. Then, a physical phenomenon happens; our scalene muscles take over and we lift our chest. We forget how to breathe. We begin to use our chest to perpetuate the breath, completely eliminating the diaphragm, and therefore lose connection.

Diaphragmatic breathing can be quite challenging in the beginning, but through conscious effort it can become second nature as in infancy. You, if like most people, most likely have not used these breathing muscles for many years. It all begins by relaxing. Particular focus needs to be drawn to expanding the abdomen and circumference of the mid lower rib cage and back. All of this should be done while keeping the chest totally stable and quiet. By doing just this one move, you will begin to make the impossible possible.

By practicing DDB 15/10 and quieting the mind, you will relearn how to relax, breathe and become more centered. Deep diaphragmatic breathing, especially coupled with meditative thought, will increase strength, increase peace, allow you to go deeper into your stretch, and increase muscle contraction ability.

This breathing exercise, by itself, can be carried out during your daily life. Gurdjeff, the great seeker of enlightenment and man's liberation from his personality, said man's hope remains in "remembering himself always and everywhere." Breathing can help you remember yourself. Breathing is something we do automatically and something we usually forget that we are doing. When we consciously control our breathing, then we can also think about remembering self. Breathing can be magical; just try going without a breath for a more than a couple of minutes.

Your body is crying out for you to heal it, and in this manual is designed to help. So quiet the mind and let's start stretching into health....

The BBD 15/10 Workout

For convenience and simplicity, I have broken the DDB 15/10 system into two separate workouts. The first consists of nine stretches focusing in on the upper back and shoulder area. The second is comprised of ten DDB stretches targeting the lower back.

One workout should take about 15 minutes to complete. Each active stretch, when done properly, incorporating the breath and mind should provide instant result of slightly increased mobility. Consistency over 4-6 weeks will have you feeling brand new. I recommend and personally try to do both workouts once a day. This ends up to be about 30 minutes a day but provides optimum results.

If you find there is a certain stretch that relieves pain in a specific problem area, repeat it as often as desired. There is no such thing as too much with this system.

Part 1

The upper back, neck and shoulders

DDB 15/10

Watch for the turning of the breath, breathe in, be aware you are filled with air, and then breathe out, being aware you're empty and need air.

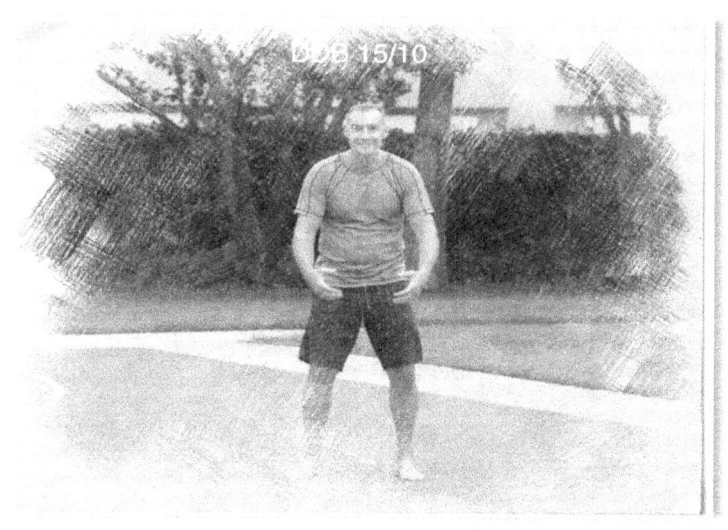

Fig 1

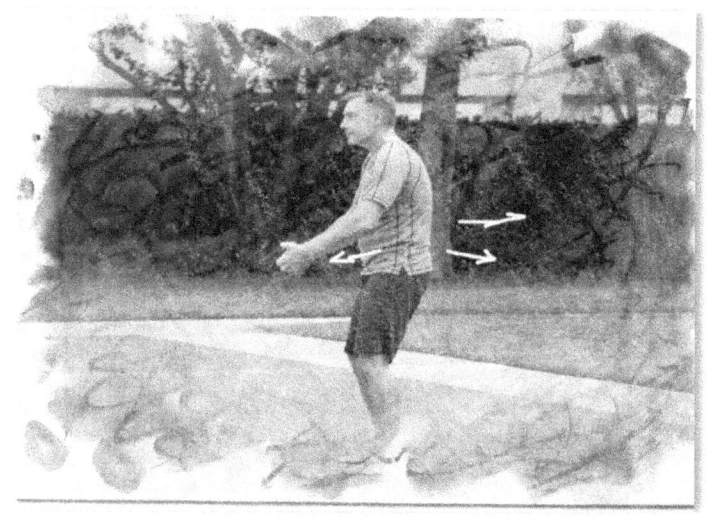

Fig 2

Deep Diaphragmatic Breath

This exercise will become automatic, and for clarification, we call it an exercise as we are learning to breathe with the diaphragm.

1. Take a stance, shoulder width, relaxed, arms open accepting air, the belly big and relaxed, allowing the low rib cage to expand with the diaphragmatic breath. This may take some body re-learning how to achieve. You were born with the ability to breathe with your diaphragm. If you are like most people, you are using your scalene muscles to lift your chest. Wrong. Be careful not to lift your chest, but focus on your lower rib cage expansion.

2. The breath, as with each exercise, is inhaled and held for fifteen seconds, filling middle and posterior of the body and not the upper chest.

3. Blow out for ten seconds (increase intensity of whatever exercise you are doing).

DDB breathing is done for every exercise shown, and is the key factor behind deep oxygenation and fascia-muscle release. Each exercise begins with deep breath held for fifteen seconds as the musculature antagonist to the stretch is contracted with 80-90 percent intensity, then released. The exercise continues with increase in intensity for additional ten seconds as the breath is released.

If you are concerned about your belly protruding, breathe with the lower part of your back and chest.

2. The Corkscrew
Internal twist straight down arm

As you pull arms towards the Earth imagine the Earth and everything you are seeing is seeing itself through your eyes and you and all are one.

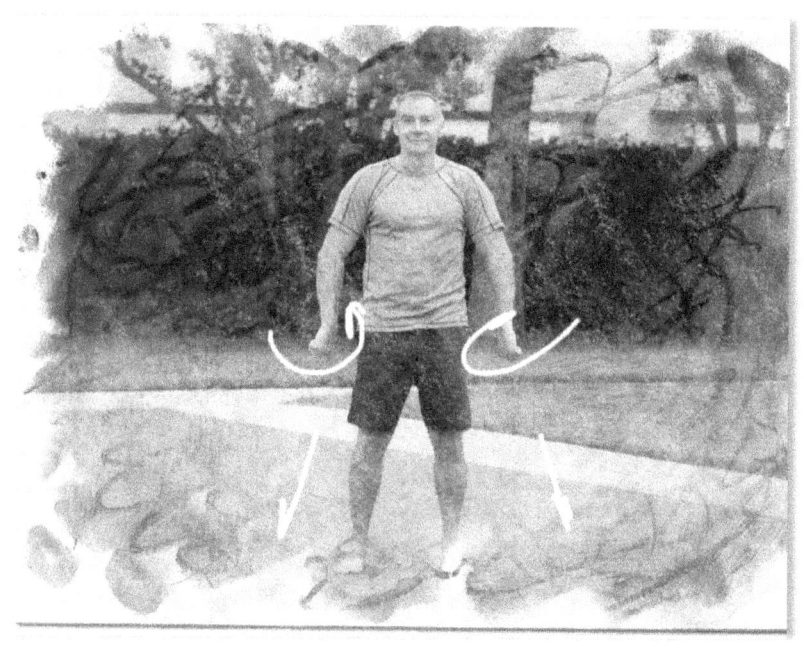

Fig 3

Internal twist, pull to earth

Internal twist straight down arm with "posterior lift."

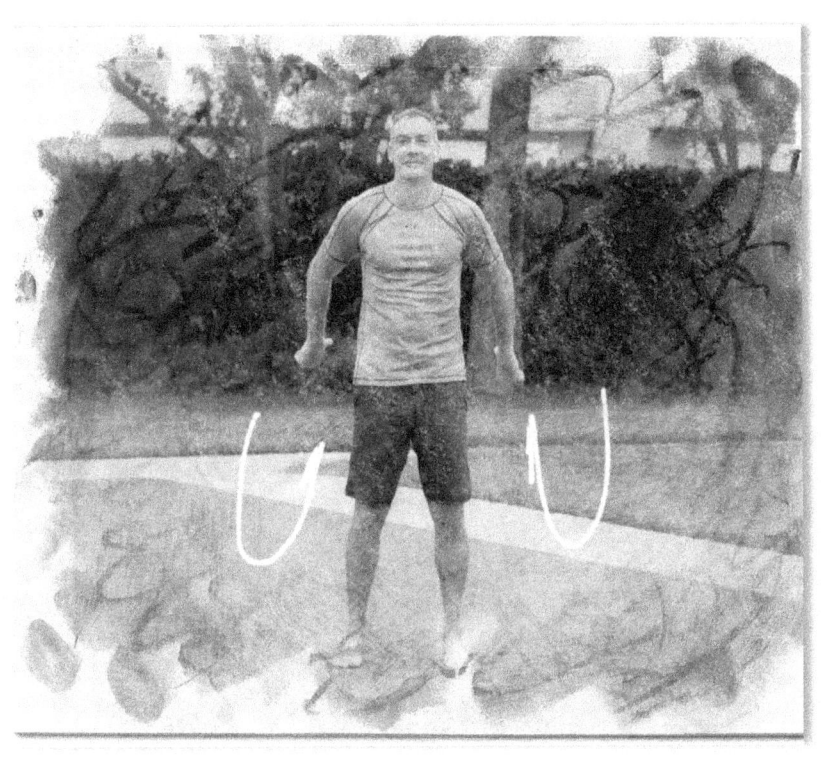

Fig 4

Internal twist straight down arm with posterior abduction

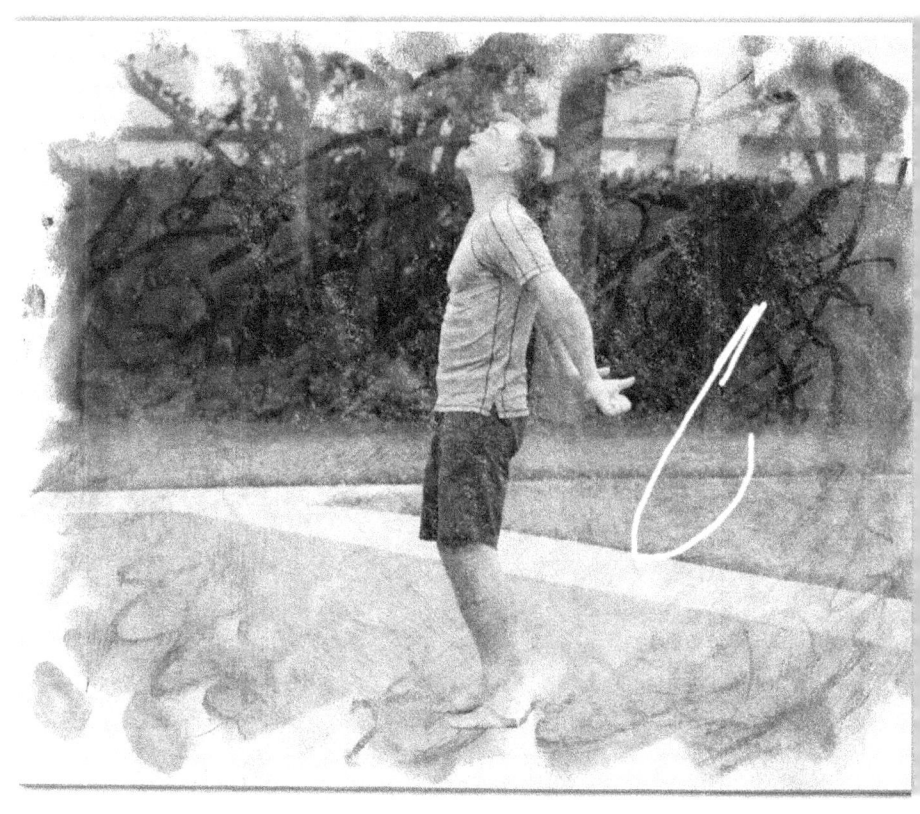

Fig 5

1. Stand with legs shoulder width apart, arms at side pointing straight down.
2. Chest up.
3. Pointing your thumbs out, begin to rotate your thumbs internally towards you until they cannot rotate any further
4. Keeping rotation, push your fists towards the ground, and elevate the chest to feel tension in the shoulders, lower, and upper arm.
5. DDB 15/10

After you have completed the straight-down arm twist, we can explore adding posterior abduction by simply beginning to lift the thumbs towards the head and away from the body.

It is important to maintain proper form and battle through the pain. The beauty about these techniques is that your body is in charge; it is your own muscle that is pulling, stretching and strengthening.

6. Take a breather and get ready to go into posterior lift.
7. Repeat steps 1-5 and keeping arms close to the body lift rotated thumbs backwards and toward the sky (see pics 4 and 5).
8. Employ DDB 15/10.

This exercise is primarily effective in helping with shoulder problems by stretching the fascia and releasing tension in the upper and lower portion of the arms. During the exercise, you may feel tension in the neck. You are welcome to rock your head into the tension getting more of a stretch in the neck region.

It is very important to remember: shoulders and the arms are pushing towards the ground as the chest is thrust forward. There should be ample to painful tension in the fascia, muscles and the skin of the whole arm and shoulder complex, including portion of the back supporting this action.

The exercise is performed under tension where the more you put into it, the more you will get out of it. The deep diaphragmatic breath is activated at the end of what one would normally deem typical effort, to take you to a whole different level of stretch and intensity. You will push towards the ground as you are twisting. When you have reached your limit, you will take a deep diaphragmatic breath and hold it for 15 seconds, where you will find a new uncharted limit and go to where you have not gone before.

At the end of the 15-second goal, you will release the air as you continue to increase the intensity of your maneuver going even further into your body. The whole idea here is to FEEL tissue stretch where you have not felt it ever before.

3. External twist, straight down arm

Accept what is. Never worry about what you cannot change; herein lies peace.

This exercise is very much like the previous as far as breathing and leg positioning are concerned.

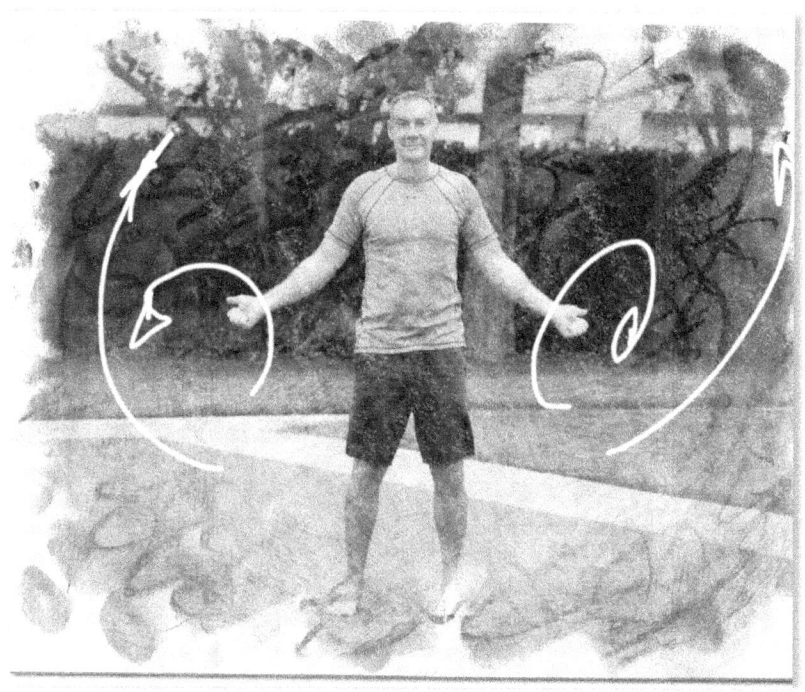

Fig 6
Front view external rotation down force

1. The arms should be straight as possible, pointing down. Some may not have the ability to get the elbows fully straight and pulling to the ground will have a greater stretch on the bicep.
2. Take a DDB deep diaphragmatic breath, pushing your shoulders and arms down to the ground as outward rotation continues.
3. Sustain for fifteen seconds as in previous and as in all exercises then release the breath, continuing to …
4. …increase intensity for additional 10 seconds of outward rotation while attempting to push the extremities to the ground.

There should be a sensation of burning in the arms and anterior shoulder if this is done properly.

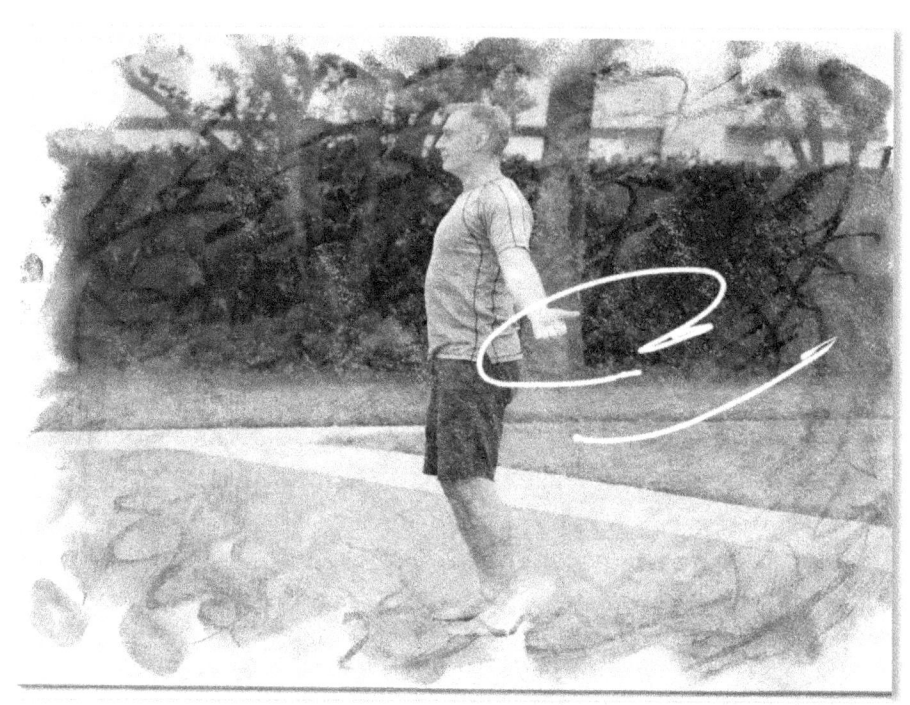

Fig 7

*Side view upper extremity,
external rotation down force.*

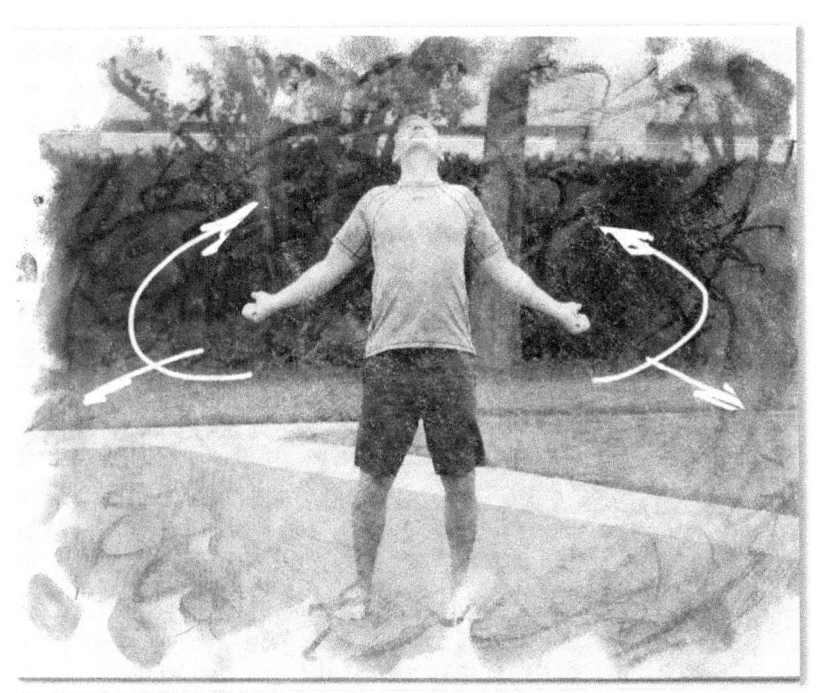

Fig 8

Front view upper extremity external rotation with abduction.

This exercise is extremely effective for opening up tight pectoral muscles, stretching the fascia in the chest and upper extremities, helping with upper cross syndrome[1], relaxing the musculature in the neck and helping with neck problems. Since most headaches are related to neck issues, practicing this maneuver may help with headaches, neck issues and shoulder problems.

This exercise is an extension of the previous external rotation.

1. As the thumbs are maximally rotated, they are also…

2. …adducting or approximating in the back, all along maintaining external rotation.

---

[1] Upper cross syndrome is when shoulders are tight causing concavity in the chest and loss of the natural curve in the neck.

Approximating your thumbs in the back will not only stretch the pectorals but will also strengthen the rhomboid and help the posture. If you stand normally in a relaxed posture and look in the mirror, you should not see the back of your hand. If you do, your pectorals may be too tight. This exercise will help correct this issue and help with most frozen shoulder problems.

If your shoulders are too frozen, you may try initially the chicken move. Bring your thumbs into your armpits and try to touch your elbows in front and back. This leads us into the chicken move.

4. The Chicken

".... either you will be killed on the battlefield and attain the heavenly planets, or you will conquer and enjoy the earthly kingdom. Therefore, get up with determination and fight."
Bhagavad Gita

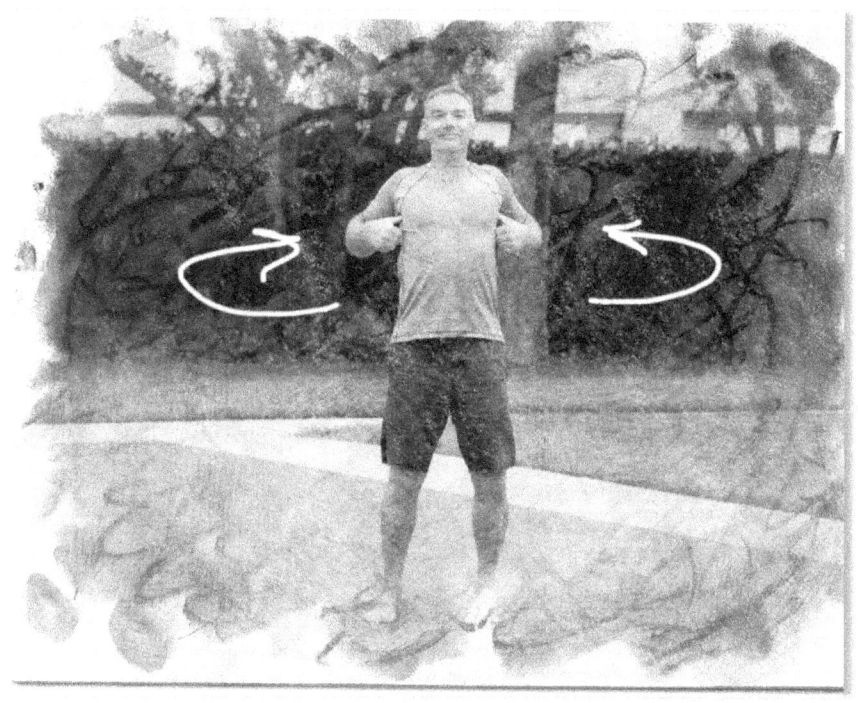

Fig 9a

1. With feet shoulder length apart, knees slightly bent, slide your thumbs up into the armpits and squeeze your elbows attempting them to touch together. (This exercise can be done with elbows touching in the front and the back.)

2. When the end point is reached where the elbows will not move any further…

3. Point elbows as high as possible.

4. Take a deep breath and hold for fifteen seconds while intensifying contracture as with all exercises, and then releasing the breath for ten as contracture intensifies, continuing to approximate, and lift elbows to the sky.

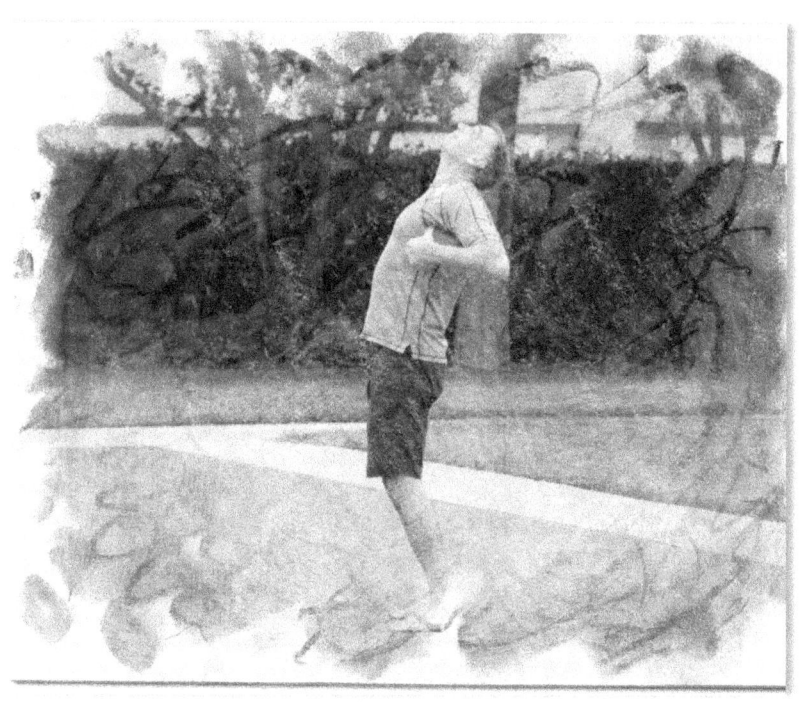

Fig 9 b

This exercise was the origin of all exercises. According to Master Tung, it was initially passed on as an ancient immediate remedy for looking thinner. As the posture changed, the shoulders lifted and corrected the posture, and the waist would get smaller by a couple of inches. It became a rave among those who were familiar with this esoteric teaching.

Recently, my very good and old friend was visiting from London with his two delightful and beautiful daughters, ages 8 and 11. What has gone unnoticed for 8 and 11 years respectively was very evident to me. Both of their spines and posture were moderately skewed. The older in particular had grown quite a bit for her age and stood at 5' 9" with a hump in her back, a major head tilt to one side, and a posture which would be not be deemed attractive for the profession of a supermodel, to which she aspired, and which, with her beauty, she could otherwise achieve.

Only after I pointed out to them the issues at hand was the so very obvious problem evident to them as well. Most people don't even notice these types of problems. We all agreed perhaps some action may be needed. I adjusted her spine and repositioned her scull with some well-placed adjustments and gave her "the chicken" exercise to do and advised her to do this on regular basis.

It may be months to years before I see her again and it will be quite interesting to see if the advice is heeded and if so the outcome of the action. Remember that for every action, there is a reaction.

5.   The Neck Stretch

In every pain there is a gain; in every problem lies a solution and a gift. Pierre Grimes

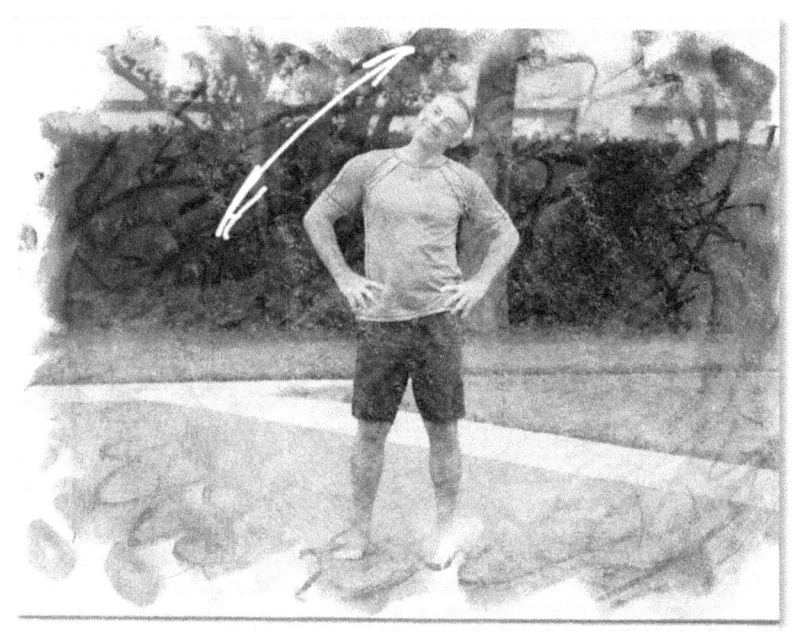

Fig 10

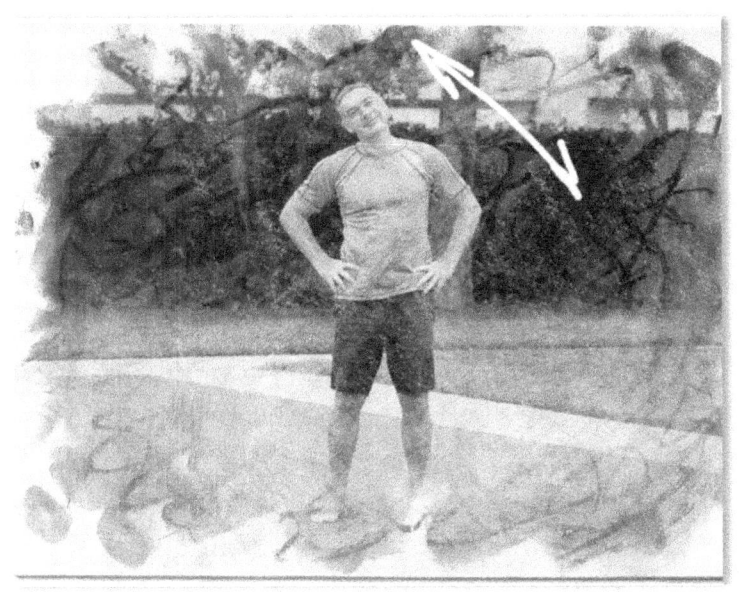

Fig 11

This is a warm-up exercise for the one to follow. Everything stays the same as previous exercises regarding feet stance and breathing.

1.   Hands are on hips and shoulders level and relaxed as the head falls to one side.
2.   Head tilts until limit is reached then inhale and hold breath for fifteen seconds and increase intensity with caution. (DDB 15/10)

The cross section diameter of a human neck bone (vertebrae) is about half inch, delicate, and in many, due to long term misalignments may be arthritic. This maneuver may be hazardous and we cannot express enough to take caution and experiment with your own abilities.

You may take a few moments to relax between these neck maneuvers; let your neck discs get in alignment before repeating. You may repeat as much of any exercise as required to optimize benefit.

6.   Chicken Wing Neck Stretch

Have great doubt, have great faith; you will figure it out,
put forth great effort to fight the illusion.
Three Pillars of Zen

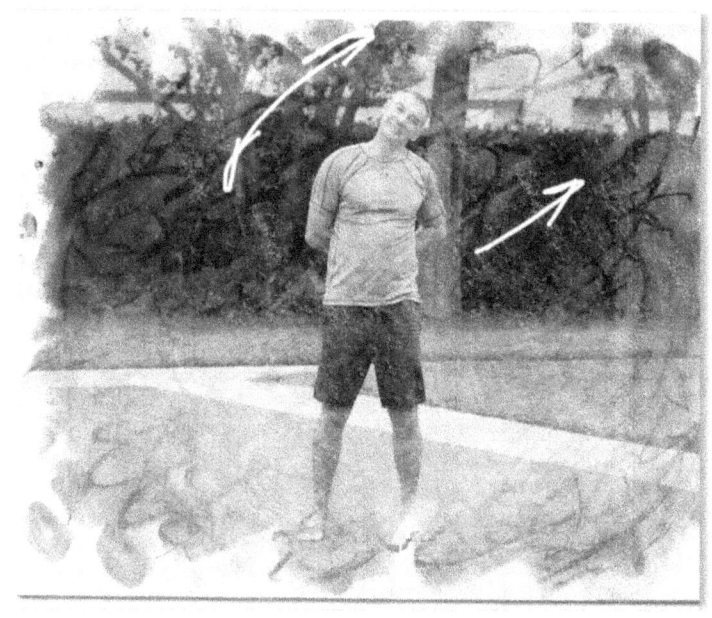

Fig 12

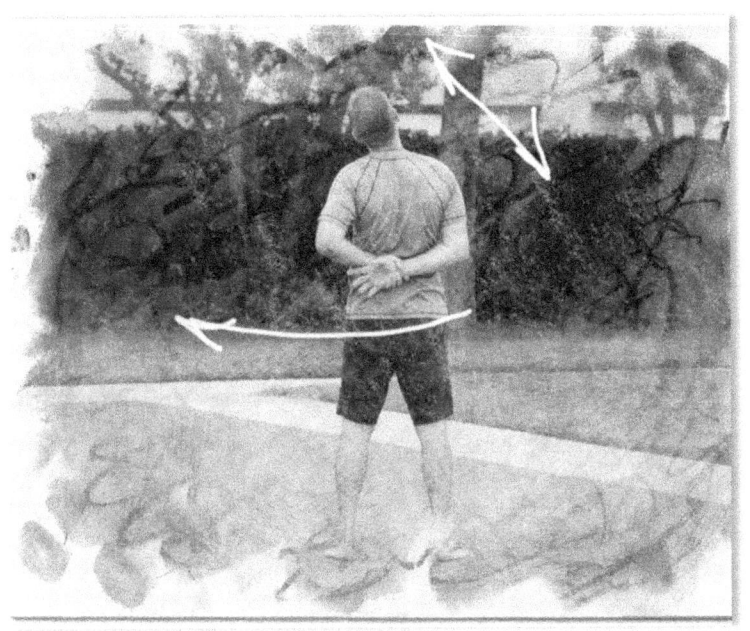

Fig 13

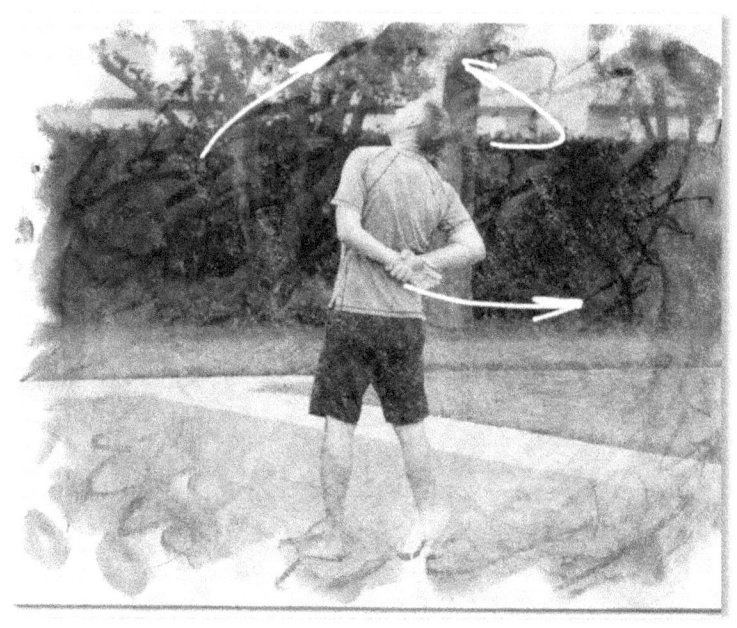

Fig 14a

3. Legs shoulder width apart.
4. Grab wrist with hand. Pull the grabbed wrist to the sky.
5. Approximate head towards the pulled wrist.
6. DDB 15/10 while stretching the side of the neck wrist is being pulled.

Take caution! Many necks are degenerating at mid-neck, so apply force according to individual ability. Repeat on other side.

7. Neck Stretch Chicken Wing with a twist

Look to the sky and find peace between the clouds like gaps between thoughts. Osho

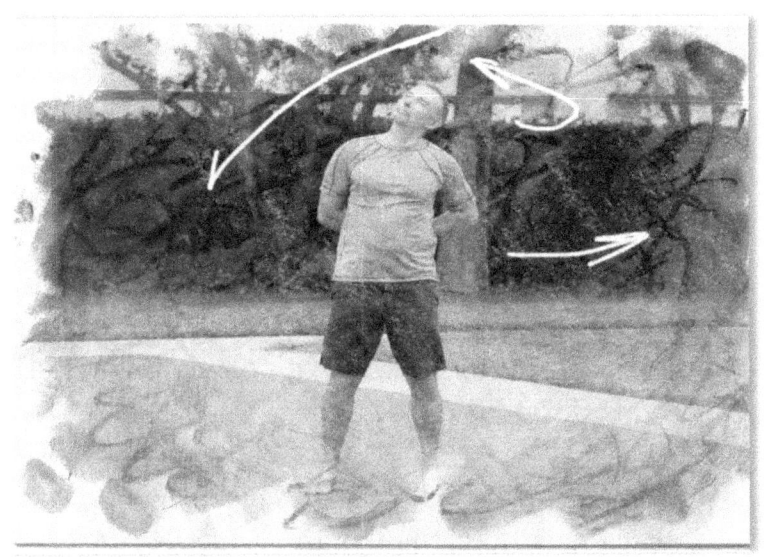

Fig 14b

Neck stretch chicken wing looking up to ipsilateral side head twist

The muscle that turns the head is called the lavator scapulae. (This may be a good Jeopardy question.) This muscle ties the tip of the shoulder blade to the back side of the head and is most active when something pretty goes by.

When the neck is stretched and the head turns this muscle gets stretched along with plenty if neck fascia, restoring flexibility to the neck.

1. Repeat exercise same as the chicken wing.
2. Turn head towards the arm which wrist is being pulled.
3. It is very important to remember the DDB is applied with every exercise.

Repeat on other side. Exercise caution and do not push through pain; just stretch.

8. The Three-Part Shoulder Buster

The difference between a winner and a loser is
one more step. Dr. Denofrio

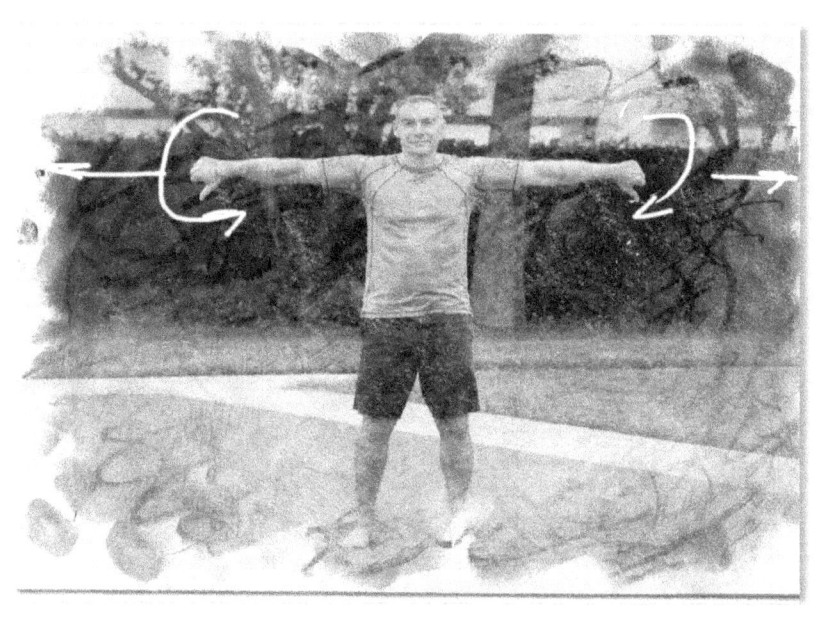

Fig 15 a
Opposing stretch down and back rotating thumbs.
Part 1

If you are like me or millions of people that could benefit from having stronger, more flexible shoulders, the following exercise is just what this doctor ordered.

Part One

1. Stand shoulder width apart as with all other exercises and
2. Elevate your arms parallel to the ground.
3. Turn your thumbs down towards the ground as if you were Caesar ordering the wining gladiator to finish his job.
4. Pull your arms directly in opposing directions with moderate intensity as if you were pulled apart by a couple of horses.
5. Twist your thumbs down and toward the back to your greatest ability, then apply the DDB.
6. When your have reached your apparent limit, take a deep diaphragmatic breath (DDB) and while holding your breath for fifteen seconds, give it your all.

7.   Pull your arms in the opposing directions while twisting your thumbs downward and posterior. When the fifteen seconds are up, blow out and continue to perform your exercise for additional 10 seconds, relaxing your breath, breathing out, and continuing to increase your contracture.

8.   You will find that you have gone an extra step that is normally not taken in an average athlete. That extra step has taken you to new limit. "The difference between winners and the losers is one extra step." If your forearms and biceps begin to burn, then you are doing your exercise properly.

Part Two

Opposing shoulder, part Deux of this exercise, is followed by bilateral arm elevation.

When you have exhausted your energy and regained your composure with the previous exercise, begin to elevate your arms as far has they will go. Your shoulders remain in the same position and act as a pivot point for your arms, which remain straight and twisted as in previous exercise. The only thing different here is that your arms are elevating to their maximum followed by the DDB protocol. When you can't go any further, apply the DDB protocol.

If this exercise is done properly, there will be burning at the shoulders and quite a bit of activity in the actual shoulder socket.

Don't forget that this exercise is also accompanied by the previous one. This means that all along while the arms are elevated to attempt to touch above the head, no matter how feeble that attempt may be, the arms are as in previous exercise pulled apart and twisted as also elevated.

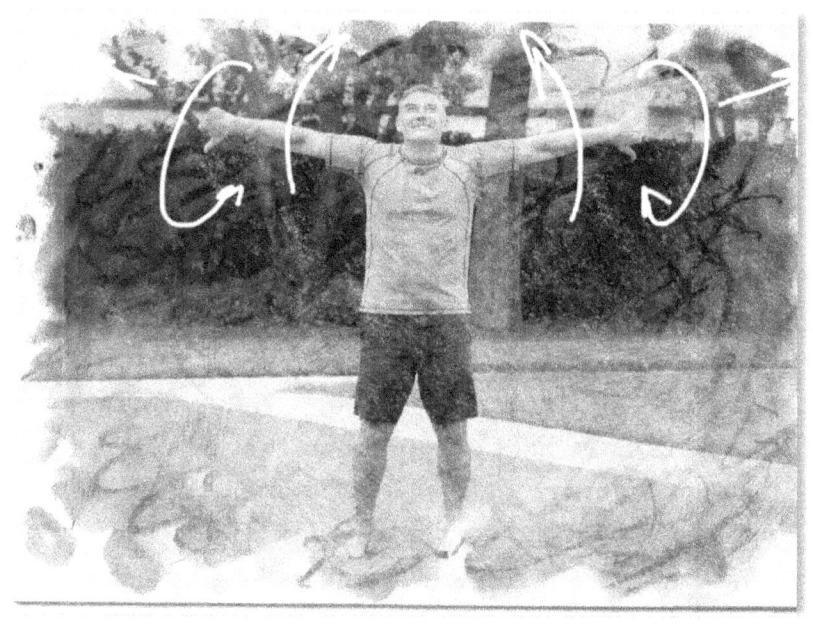

Fig 15b

Twist pull and elevation. Part 2

This leads us into part 3…

Part Three

Part three of the shoulder buster is a continuation of part one. The only difference is that in part three, from arm parallel to the ground position as in part two, the arms are pulled back all the way, utilizing all the rules aforementioned in part one, but instead of going up as in part two, we go backwards, attempting to approximate our hands behind. When we reach our perceived limit, we activate our DDB system, taking the exercise to the ultimatum contracture our antagonist muscles will allow. It is quite important to maintain the proper form throughout all of our exercises and particular attention here is paid to maintaining arms parallel to the ground.

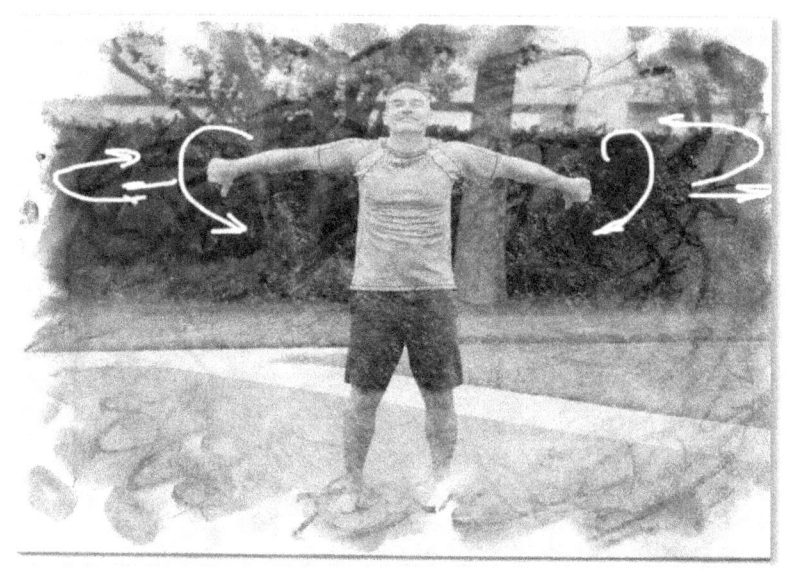

Fig 15 c
Shoulder buster part three, posterior pull

Shoulders are pulled back and arms are at a parallel to the ground level. It always helps to go through all of these exercises looking in the mirror to maintain the proper form.

No effort, no gain. We will discuss the mind behind the mind at the end of the manual.

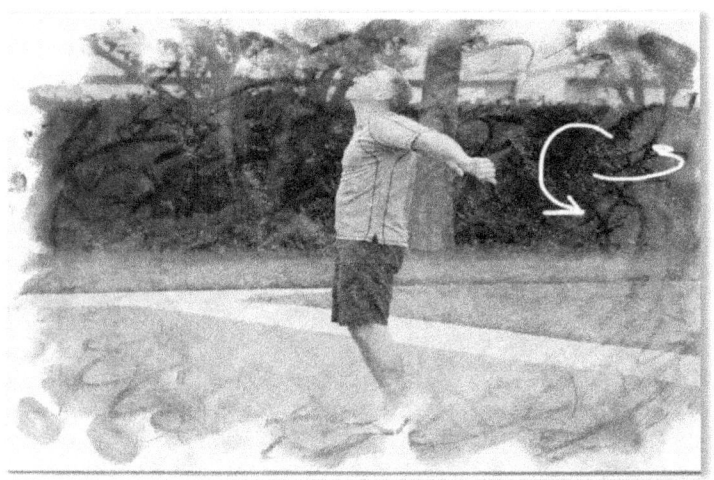

Fig 15 d *Part three, side view*

Here the arms should be parallel to the ground and pulled back, using the DDB system.

9. Part Three, Shoulder Buster Reversed

What is it actually that is doing this exercise?
Pierre Grimes

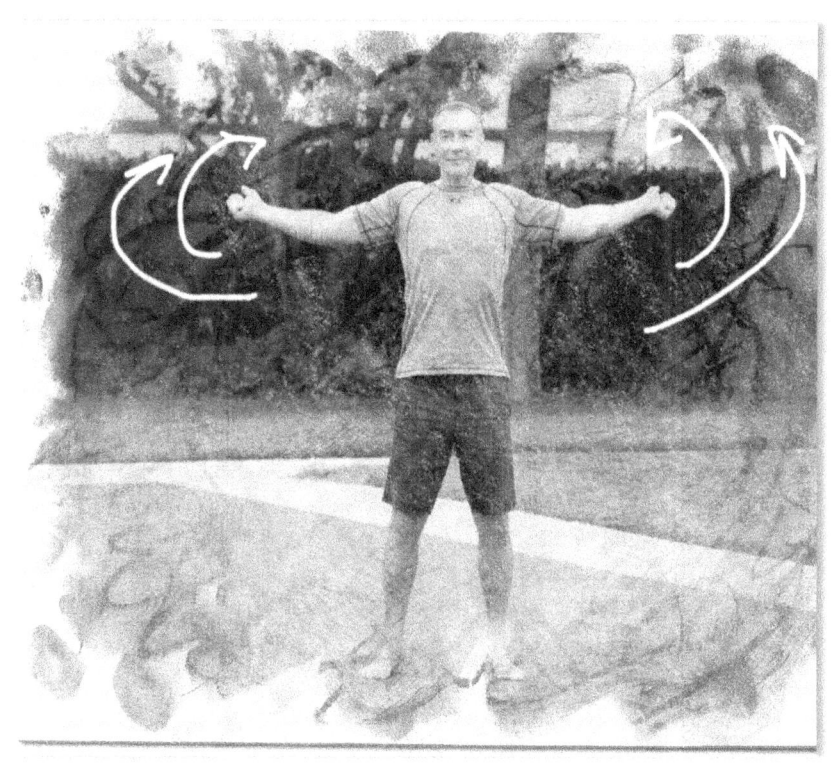

Fig 16 a

"He lives" order, with arms pulled apart and thumb
twisted up and back.

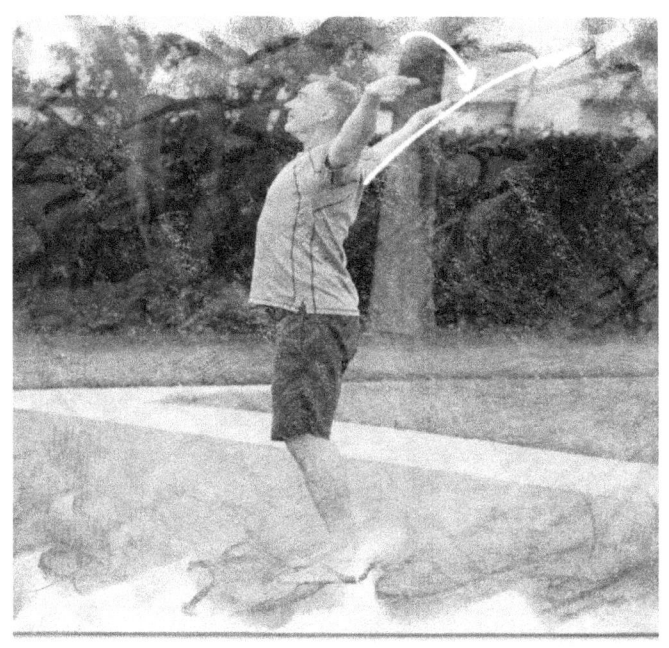

Fig 16 b

.....and then adding arms pulled back.

This set is exactly the same as the thumbs down for a "Caesar's Kill Order." This one is a "Caesar's Live Order," thumbs up with a twist. Arms are pulled apart and twisted. DDB system takes it to the extreme.

10. The Shoulder Buster Variant

The mind may just truly be all that really is.

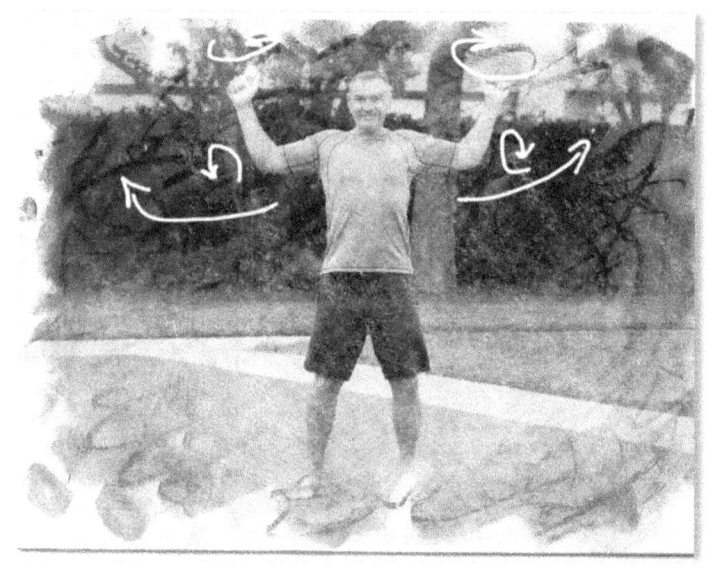

Fig 17a

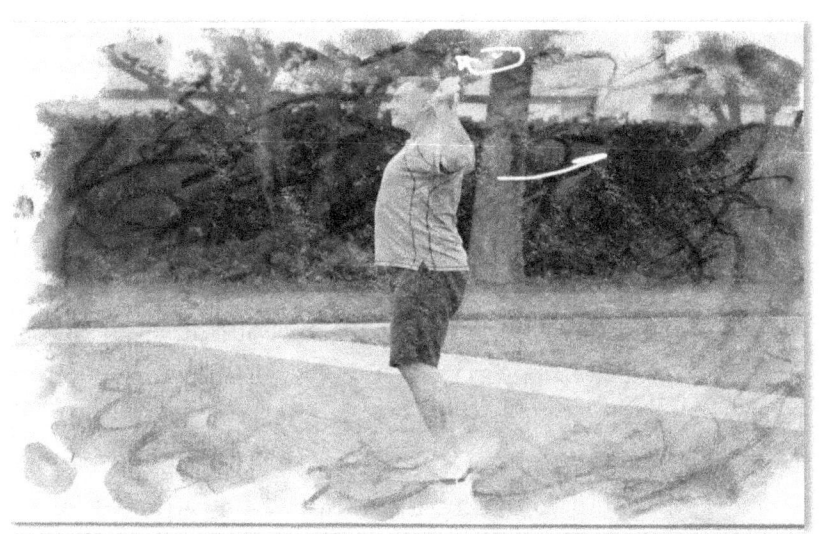

Fig 17b

1. Shoulder external rotation is performed with elbows and arms at 90 degrees.

2. With arms parallel to the ground with elbows at 90 degrees, rotate your arms to the hilt; then begin the DDB system.

3. Shoulders are relaxed, with the upper arm parallel to the ground and with elbows at 90 degrees, try to bring your forearms posterior.

4. The second part of this exercise involves continuing to stretch your arms at a 45 degree angle caudal, or to the sky, all along, approximating your thumbs behind your back.

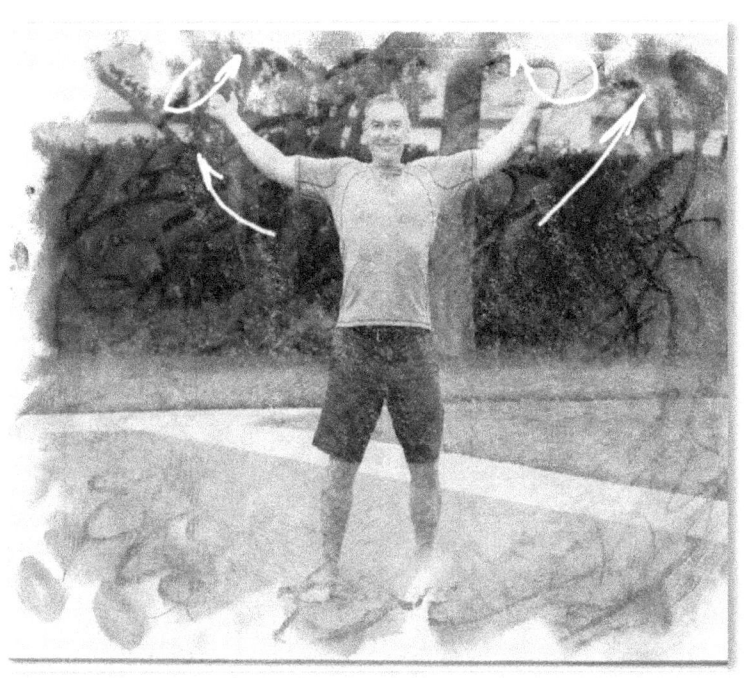

Fig 17c

External rotation with 45 degree caudal
posterior extension.

11. The 45-degree Opposing Extension

Accept death as part of life and look forward to your new suit as liberation.

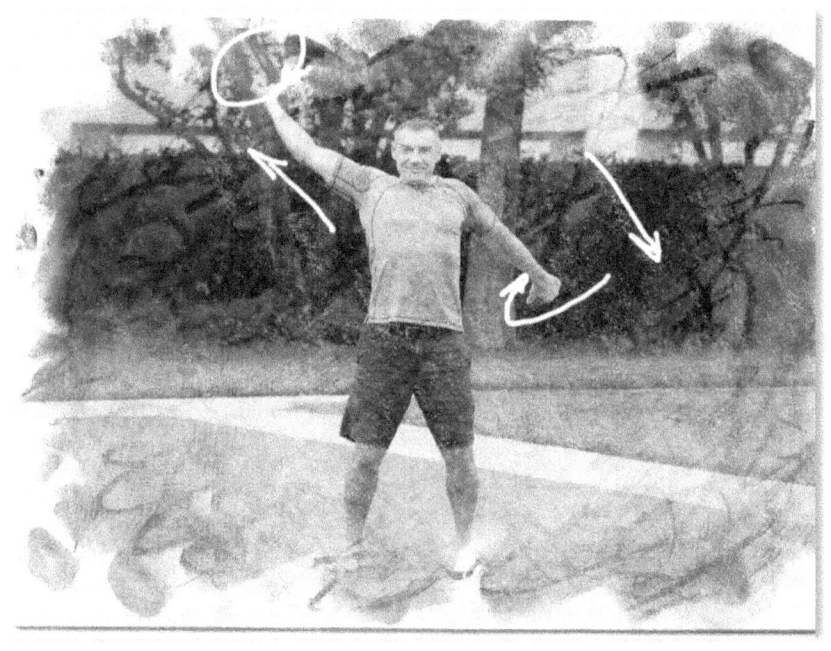

Fig 18a

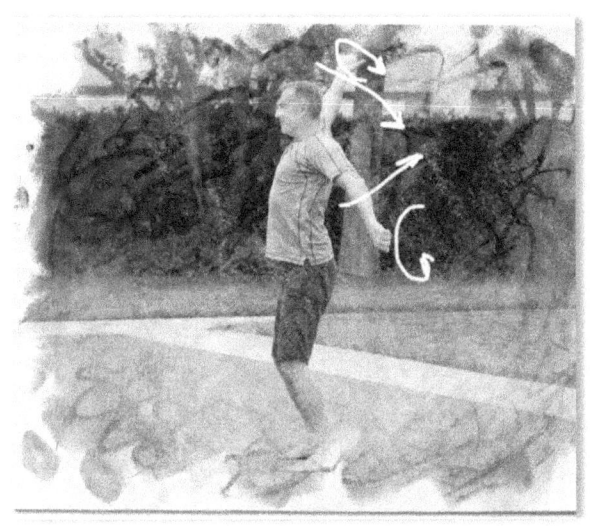

Fig 18 b

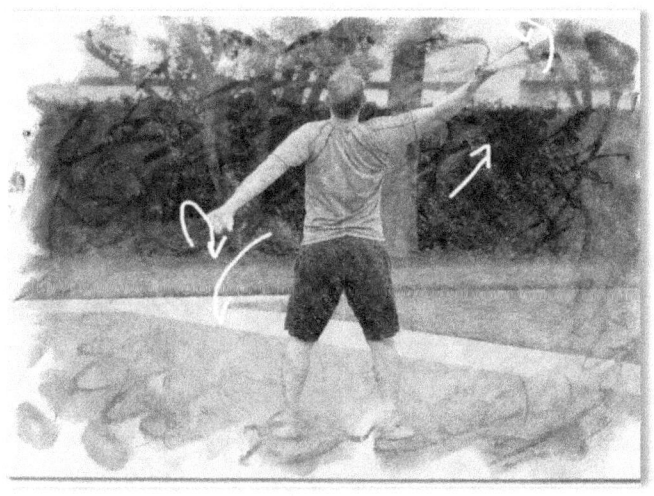

Fig 18c

A variant from the previous exercise, twist and extend and pull posterior as arms are pulled apart in opposing angles.

DDB here goes without saying, as it does for all other exercises.

12. Double back fist up and lift.

Where is the Mind?

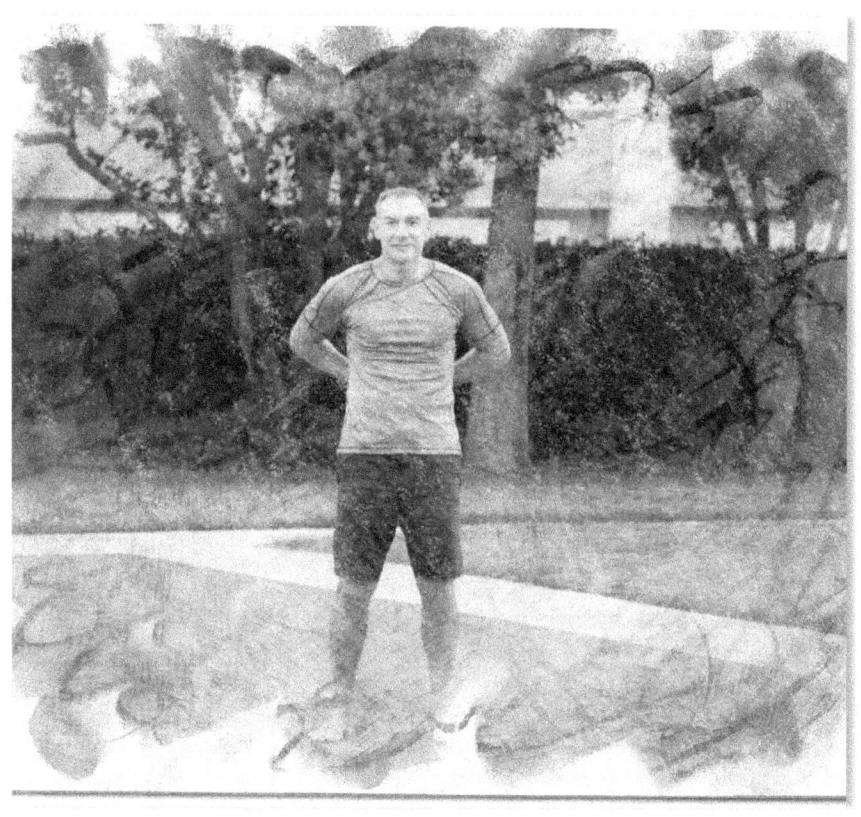

Fig 19a

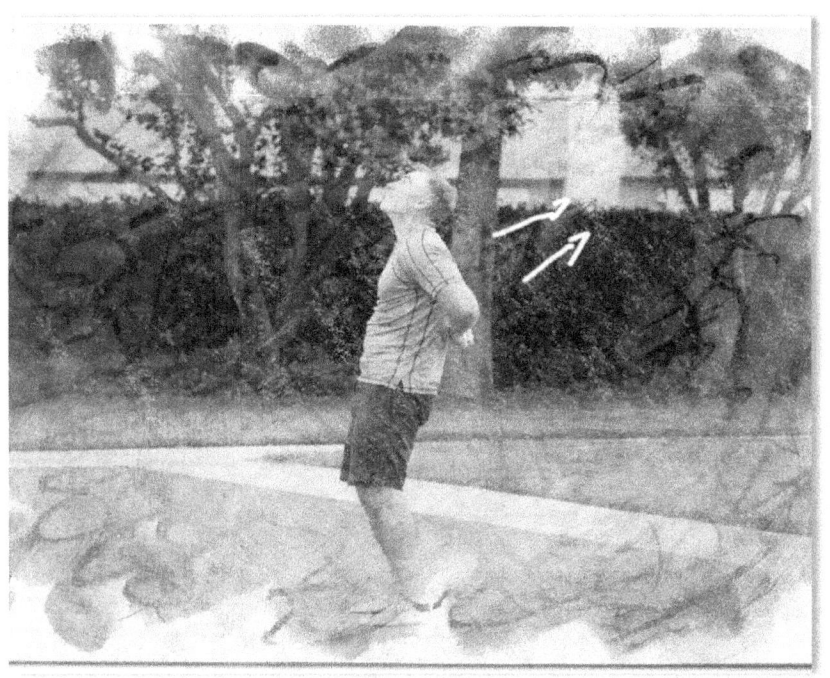

Fig 19b

This just may be the very first exercise I began doing to unfreeze my shoulder. I deem it the mother of all exercises, for in me, it was this very motion that was the most limited, exuded the most pain, and so it was the motion that got the ball rolling for developing all the others.

The stance and the breathing are standard, as it was for all the previous exercises.

1. You begin by testing how far up the back your fist can go, and if you are like most people, it may be difficult to get one arm as high as the other or both.
2. With your feet shoulder length apart, bring both fists behind the back as far up as they will go.
3. DDB as you begin to elevate your fists up the back and…

4.   ...AWAY from the torso and up the back with as much intensity as possible for 15 seconds, and then increase intensity for another 10 seconds as the breath is released.

Elevate the head to maximize intensity as fists are thrust in the upward and away motion.

The Bottom Half

Watch for the turning of the breath
when inhaling and exhaling.

We have just completed the upper body and are now going to discuss the bottom part.

The DDB system applies here as it does for all exercises as the basis for stretching the fascia, increasing energy and strengthening the whole constitution.

We begin the first exercise called the "Bend Over" with the DDB system and the original stance as in the very first picture.

13.   The Bend Over

Victim energy lives within when you give it life.

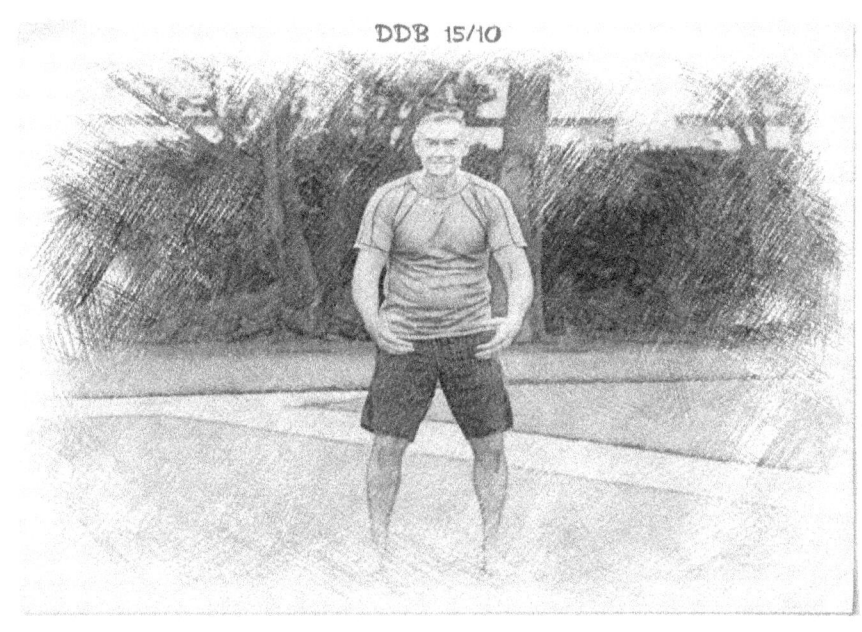

Fig 20 a

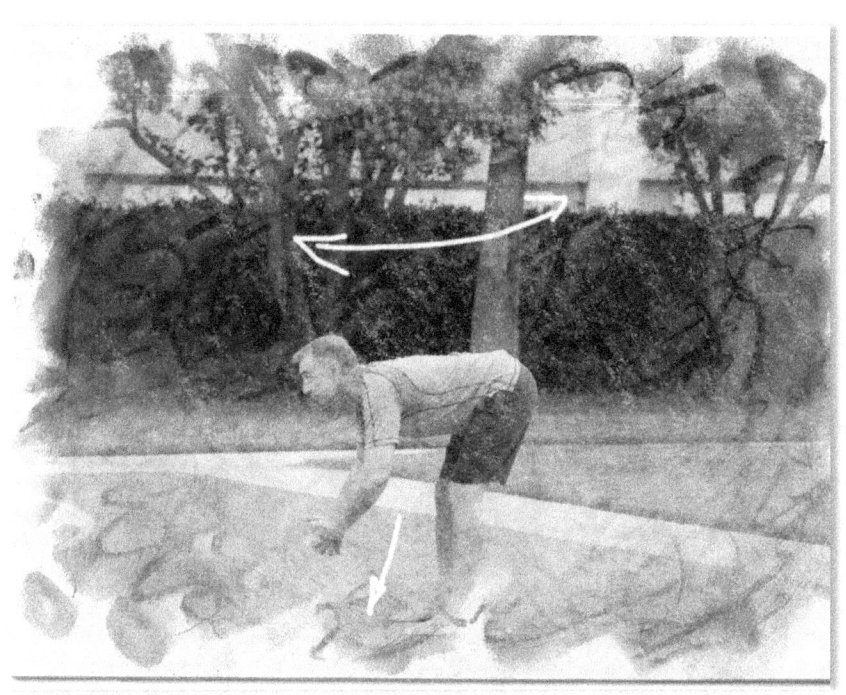

Fig 20 b

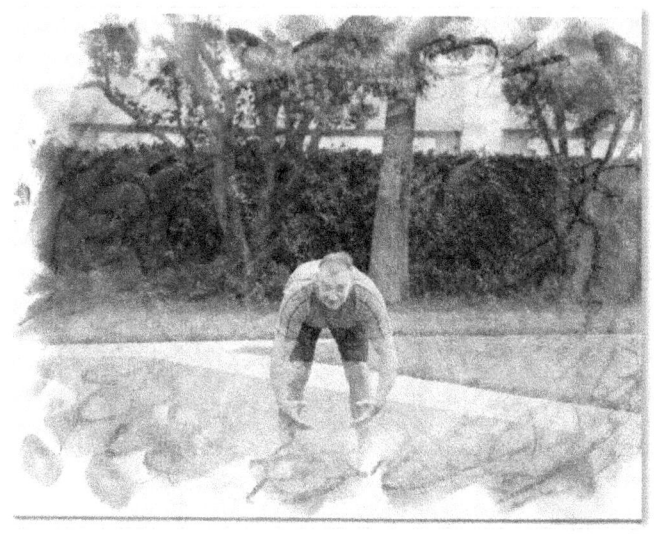

Fig 20 c

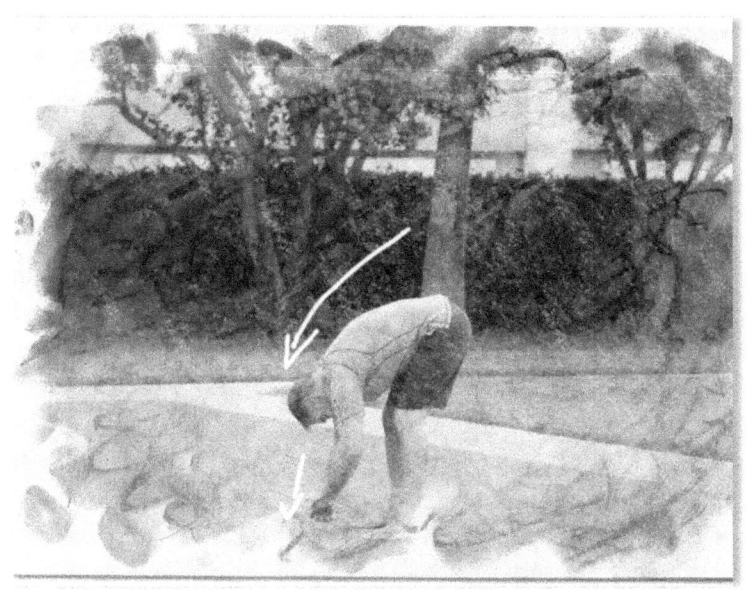

Fig 20 d

1. With a DDB system, big air belly.

2. Begin to bend at the waist with legs straight and the back with lordotic curve. DDB means you are now bent over, arms hanging to add weight, and using gravity and core strength.

3. Attempting to touch the head to the ground, keep the back arched back and force the butt up in the air like you don't care for full 15 seconds, then release the air and allow the torso to fall to the ground, approximating head to the floor for additional 10 seconds, never letting up on the intensity. This exercise offers tremendous relief to musculature in the low back, letting go of much tension.

To maximize release in the legs, I instruct my patients to do it with feet in three positions: neutral, pigeon-toed and Charlie Chaplin. See pictures on the following pages.

Foot positioning

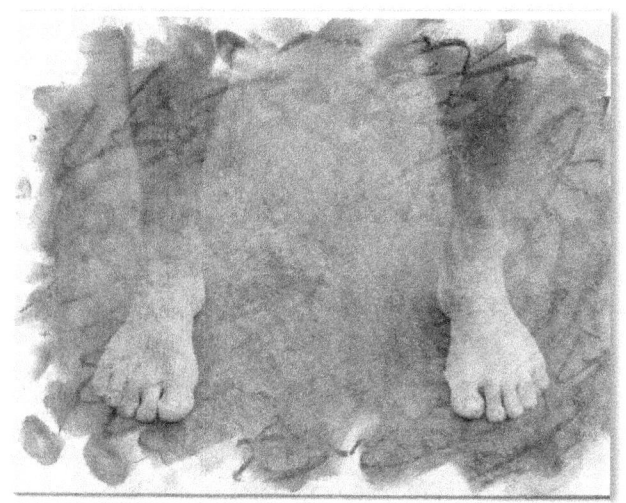

Fig 21 a

The Neutral

Foot positioning in this exercise is quite important. The neutral is the most stable and gives a general hamstring stretch which releases the pelvis and take a quite bit of tension in the low back.

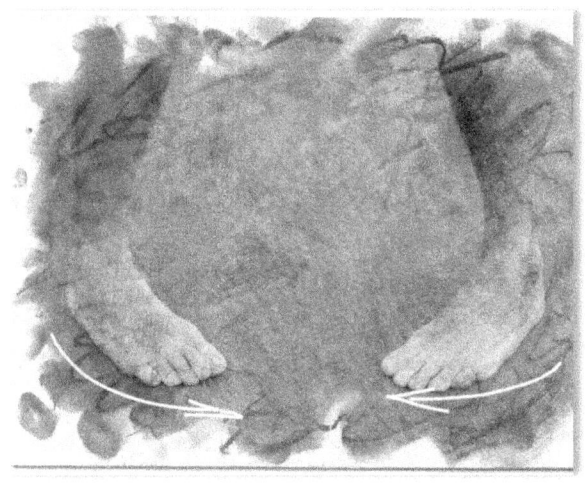

Fig 21 b
The Pigeon Toe

The pigeon toe will stretch the fascia outside of the legs where most people with low back problems will have tension. Practice the bend over with all three foot positions daily and watch for a miraculous low back recovery as many of my patients have.

Rotate between neutral, pigeon and Chaplin as needed to maximize results. Each foot position will be a benefit and will maximize benefit.

The pigeon in bend over is tremendous on releasing all sort of tension that would normally be difficult to reach.

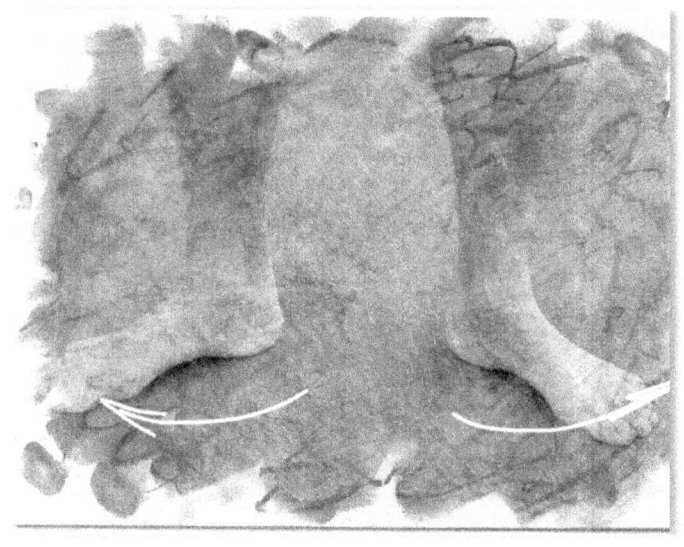

Fig 21c

The Charlie Chaplin

Continuous DDB system employed on all foot positions in continuous circle creates most benefit.

14. The Bend Back

Mind is a like an untrained dog, reflexive, reactive, and loves sniffing things of gross nature.

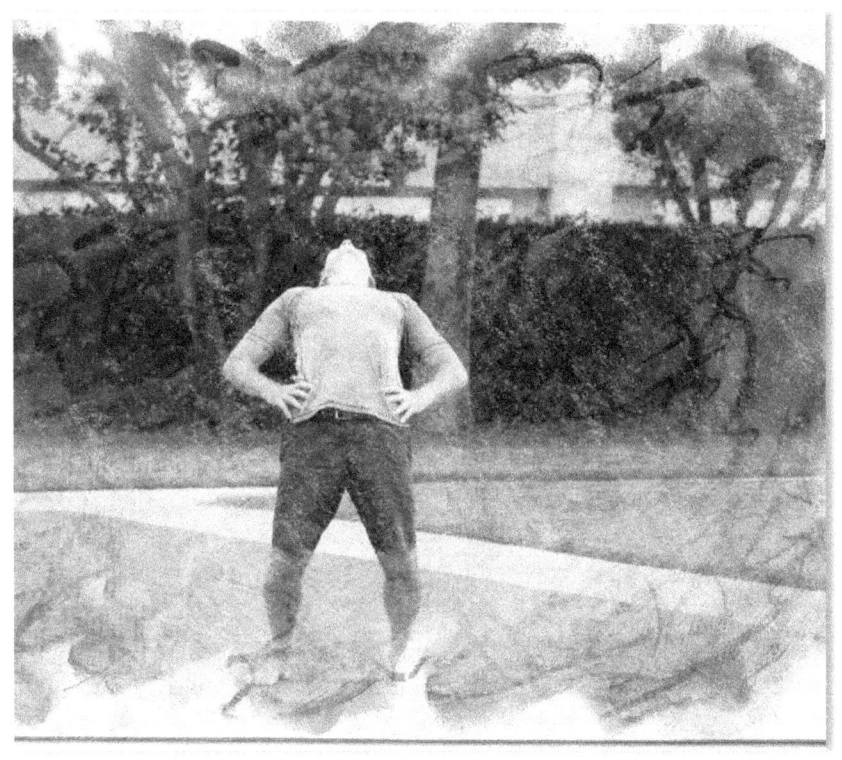

Fig 22

Proceed with caution.

To counter the effects of bending forward, we must bend back.

1. So far, the stance is all the same, with legs shoulder width apart.

2. The hands are on the hips for balance, we extend all the way back, and then go into our DDB, forcing the back to go back and further back than ever before.

This exercise is tremendous for back issues and it can be so powerful, yet caution must be exercised. When we bend back, we are actually moving our discs to a different position in relationship to bones. This can be quite dangerous and you may want to consult a competent chiropractor that has your X-ray to assure your lower back is in good shape to do this maneuver.

When we sit, our bones shift and the posterior of the bone must flare and allow the disc to move; otherwise, you would be sitting with your back arched. Actually, this is an ideal way to sit if just for that purpose alone, to maintain a good bone-disc relationship.

When we slouch, we establish a very poor bone-disc relationship and when we stand up straight, we hope it all falls back in place. In humans, sitting with the back arched may not always be the case.

The human vertebrae complex has been designed for a four-legged animal. When we humans stand, bones may slip out of alignment.

In any case, proceed with caution.

As you bend back, see if your back will allow you to go back. If at first it feels sketchy, you may skip this exercise and go to some other, and when things are a bit more lubed up and you feel more confident, then revisit.

Proceed with caution and consult your chiropractic physician prior to attempting this maneuver.

15. The Lunge

Remember yourself at all times.   Gurdjieff

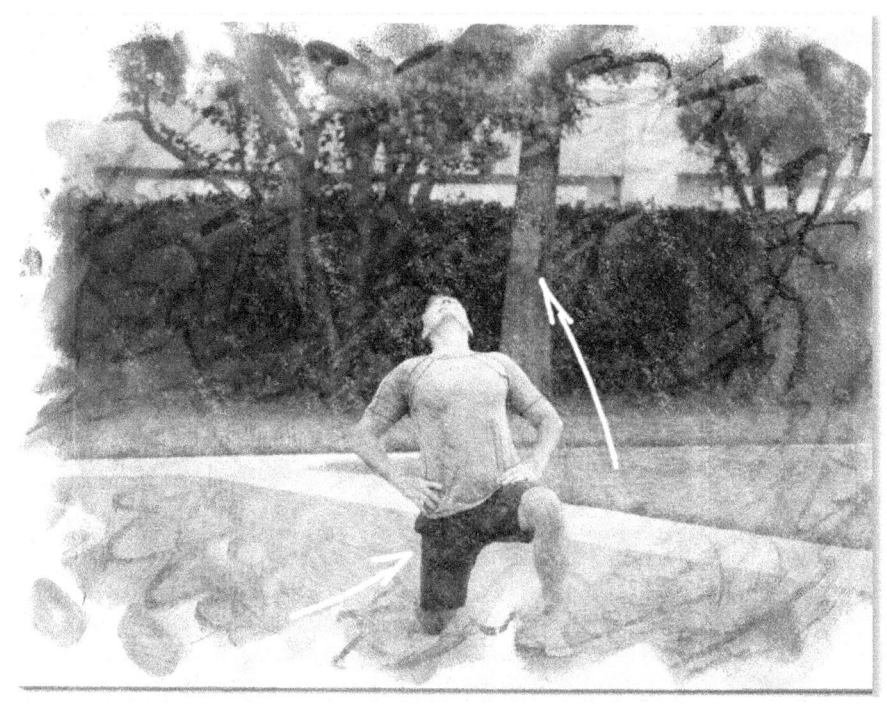

Fig 23a

This is an ultimate quad stretch for the leg with the knee on the ground.

1. Your legs are shoulder width apart, the quad being stretched has the knee on the ground, and the other leg is at 90 degrees in a lunge position.

2. The quad being stretched is in its maximum stretch position.

3. DDB system is applied, where we take a deep diaphragmatic breath.

4. Put the torso in a posterior extension while holding the breath for 15 seconds; then release and continue the stretch for an additional 10 seconds, maximizing the fascia muscle stretch.

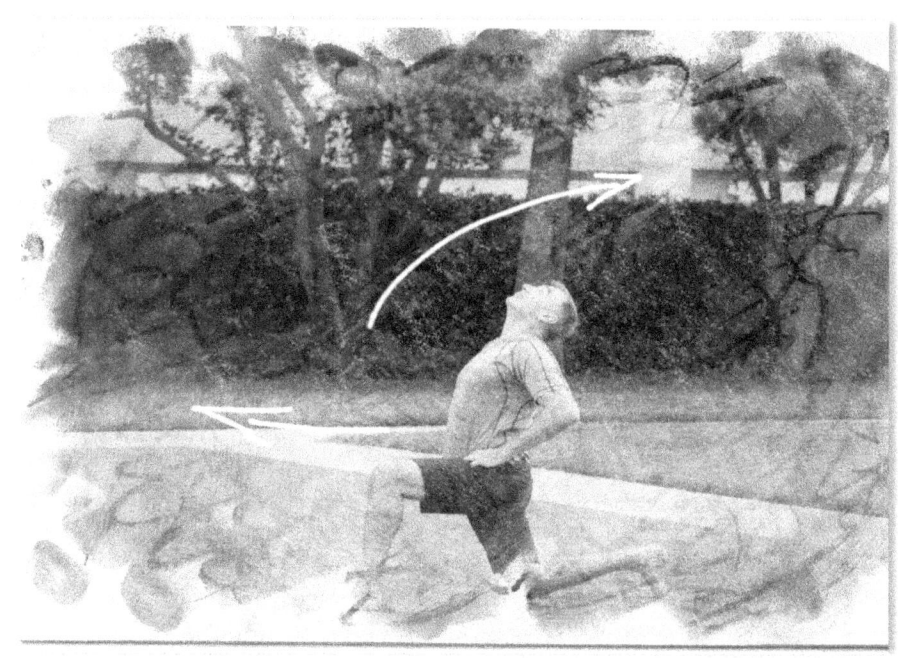

Fig 23 b

Quad stretch side posture, DDB

Here we are looking for two things. One is stretching the quads and contracting the back and the other is what is occurring with the bones of the low back. This can be a very beneficial for the low back, but also heed caution and don't overdo it.

16. The Torso Twist

Smile to remember to remember yourself.

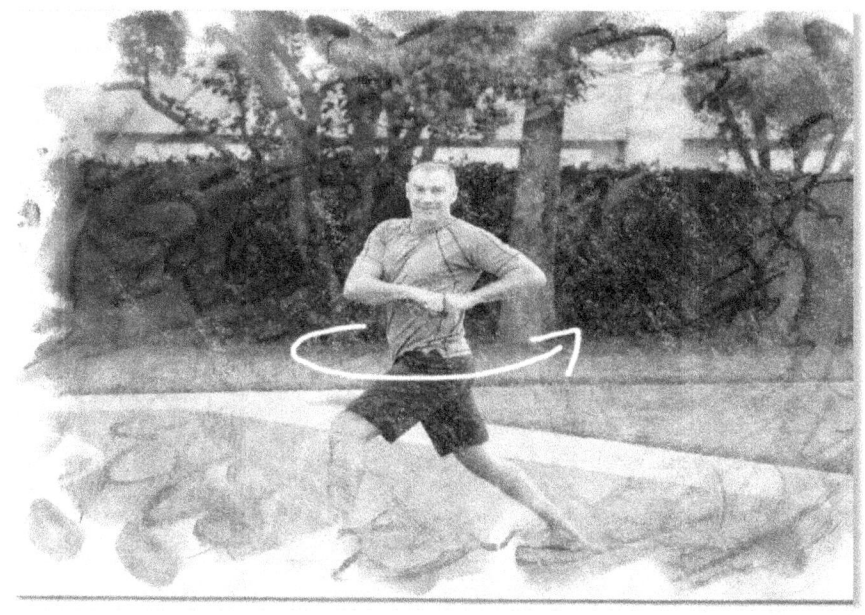

Fig 24

The torso twist is best performed after completing the lunge as an offshoot.

1. Legs are shoulder width apart, in a lunge stance. Here again you are working with your own body and your ability.

2. Use fists instead of a closed hand to push the opposing elbow to increase the torso stretch.

3. DDB system is deployed as quadratus lumborum, the four big muscles in your low back, are stretched to the hilt. Twist till you cannot go further.

4. DDB is held for 15 seconds as intensity of exercise increases and continues to increase for additional 10 seconds as breath is released.

This exercise can be repeated as needed symmetrical from side to side. Switch legs and twist to the opposite side as needed, or until the stiff bones in the back "let go" or click in place. Use caution and a little common sense; don't push it.

17. The Side Bend

Duality is a contradiction to knowing thyself.

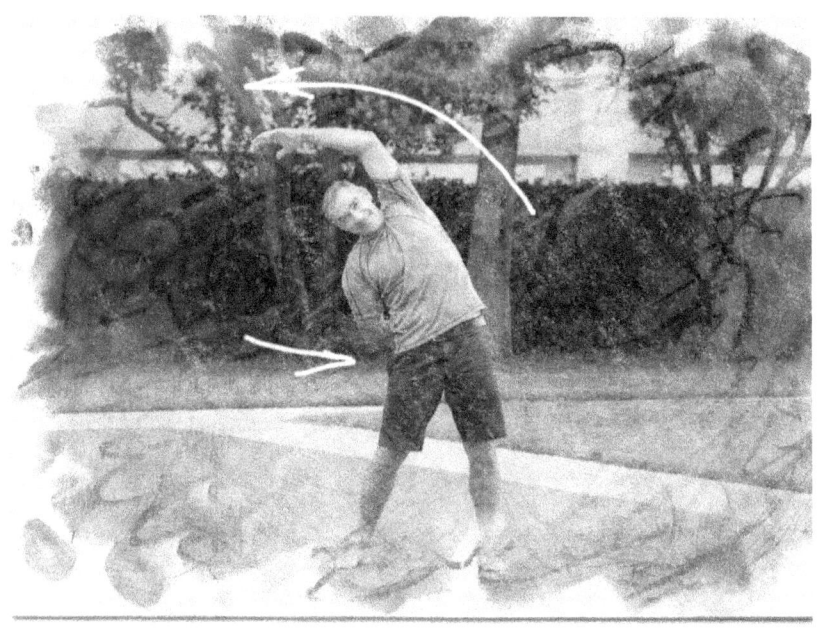

Fig 25

Legs are shoulder width apart.

1. With one arm above head and one behind the body, diametrically oppose force along fingers to your maximum stretch.

2. Reach for the sky or a star, feel it pull your arm out of the socket, then bend and feel the tension all along the side from the hip to the tip of the pinky, pulling in the opposite direction with the arm behind your back.

3. Take your tension as far as it will go, and take a DDB using the 15-second, 10-second rule. Think fascia and feel all the tension and stretch into it.

18. The Split and Sit

Buddha said, whatsoever you do, do with full consciousness.

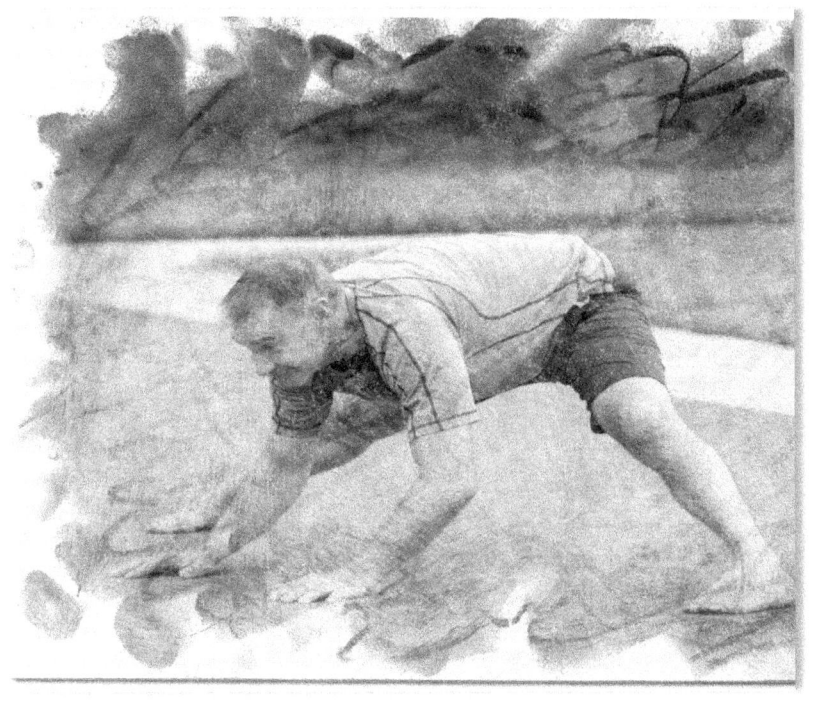

Fig 26 a

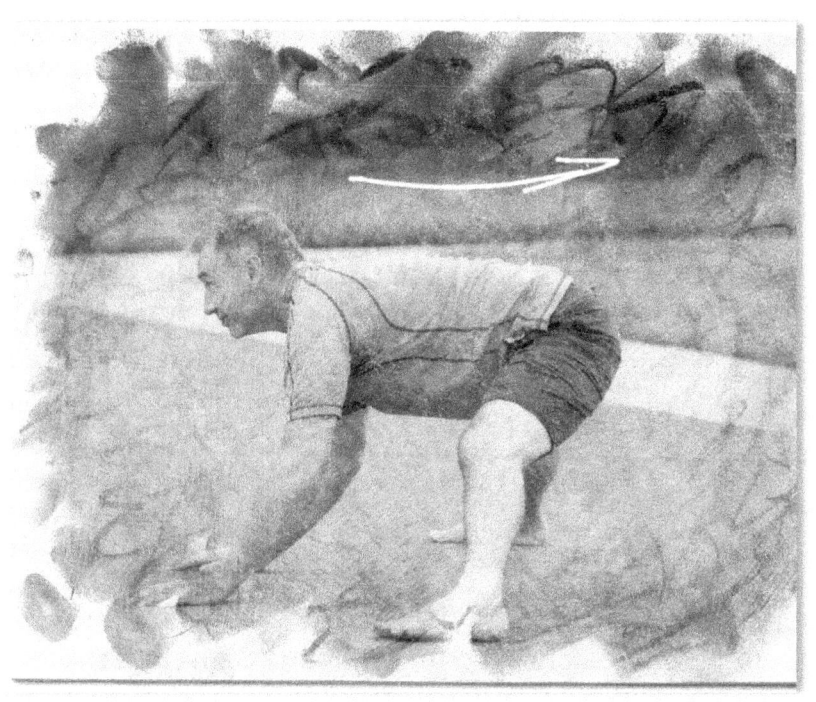

Fig 26 b

The Split and Sit pelvic stretch

Lots of low back issues stem from the pelvis and tight upper leg muscles. Inevitably after every leg workout, the low back becomes very susceptible to injury, aches, tension, or some sort of discomfort. Stretching the fascia and deep surrounding pelvic tissue will increase mobility and provide freedom in the low back, allow for the bones to move, and "pump" the discs. The motion induced in the discs will allow for the nerves to free up, reduce pain, and allow for the "juice of life" to flow to your organs.

1. Spread your legs using the floor with your hands to guide your feet out until you begin to feel you have reached the end of your stretch.
2. Take a DDB and for 15 seconds
3. Attempt to push your butt down. Breathe out and continue for additional 10 seconds.

19. Wall Reverse Split

Imagination is more important than knowledge. For knowledge is limited, whereas imagination embraces the entire world, stimulating progress, giving birth to evolution. Einstein

Knowledge is based on your programing, which is usually wrong.

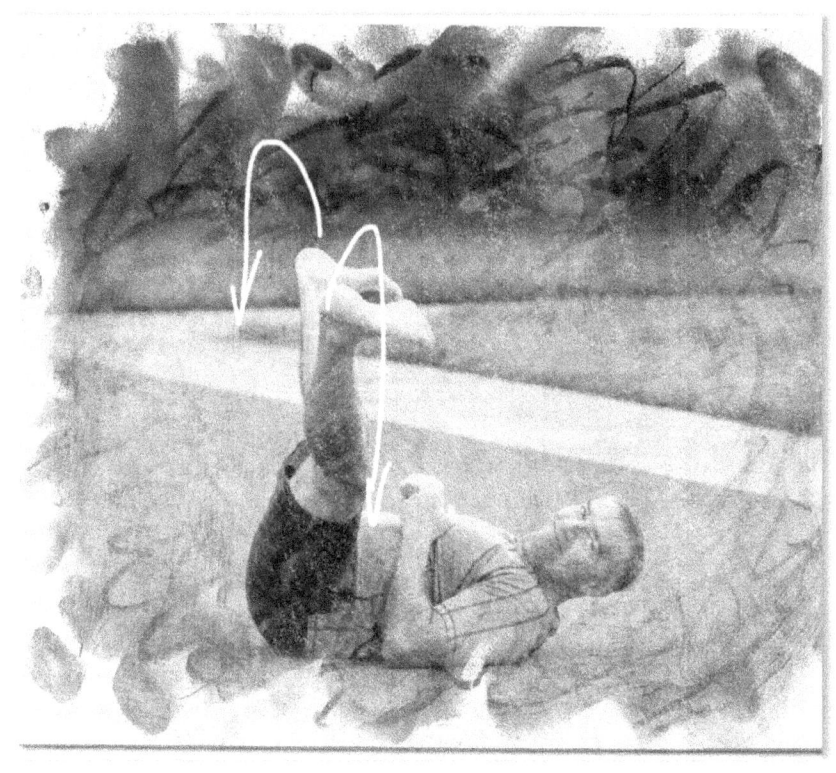

Fig 27

A variant to the split and sit is a wall reverse split.

Here we are using a special see-through wall so you can get a visual. Legs are straight; we are using gravity and the DDB system to exercise.

1. Slide your butt all the way up against the wall.
2. Lie down on the floor and allow your legs to fall apart from each other.
3. Here a regular stretch would be to allow the gravity to open your legs. This is a great stretch and it can turn into one awesome exercise when at the end point you take a ...
4. DDB and apply the 15-10 rule. With legs in the air, take a DDB and for 15 seconds, attempt to open your legs further; then blow the air out and for additional 10 seconds, intensifying abduction as the breath is released.

The wall reverse splits are actually best when used against the wall or without the wall as depicted in the picture. This can be done in a seated position, using abductors to open the legs while using the DDB system 15/10 system. It works as a great strengthening workout on groups hardly used.

20. The Legs and Back

When the perception is understood, what can be real in the unreal realm?

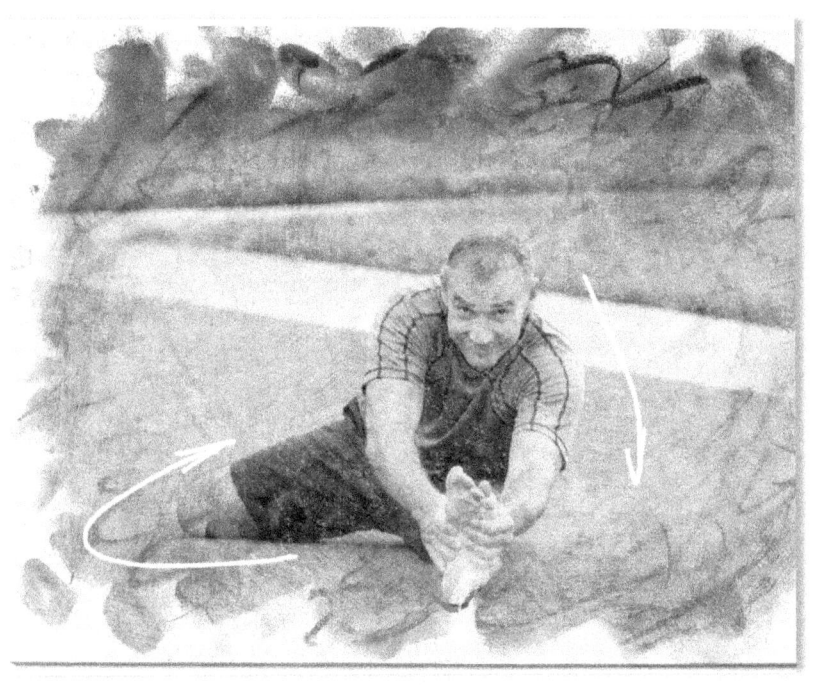

Fig 28 a

1. From the split, we can twist towards the left.

2. Sit and grab a leg, stretching the hamstrings and the quad on the opposite side. This seems to be stretching the legs, but the idea here is to stretch the fascia in the back of the torso as a focal structure.

3. Grab the front foot in the split take a DDB.

4. Bend the head down feeling the fascia in the neck and tightness in regions of the torso.

5. Hold breath for 15 seconds as you actively release and stretch into the tight regions of the neck and back.

6. Continue to increase intensity for 10 seconds more as the breath is released.

It's perfectly OK to move the head side to side to communicate with your fascia, as your tension lets go.

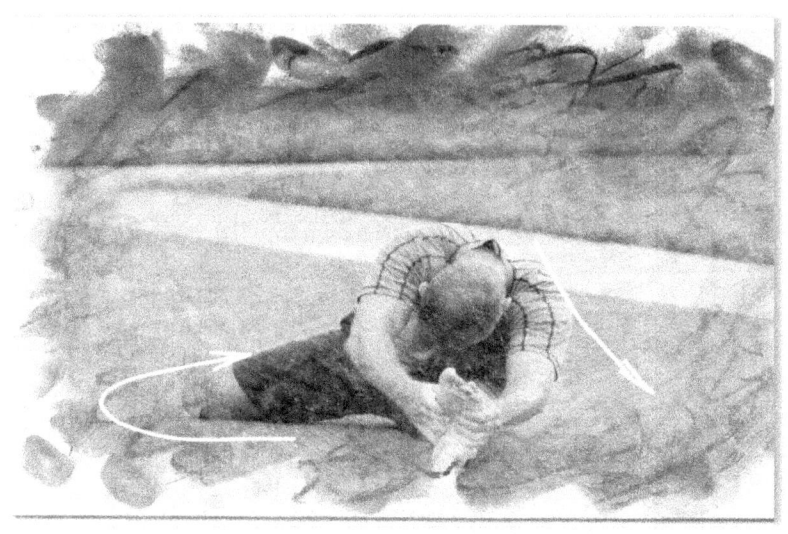

Fig 28 b

Start with the head up, then bring your head down to stretch the neck and back fascia.

Bring the head down during the DDB hold for 15 seconds; then increase intensity for an additional 10 seconds as you release the breath.

21. Double Ham and Back

Human is the only bored animal.

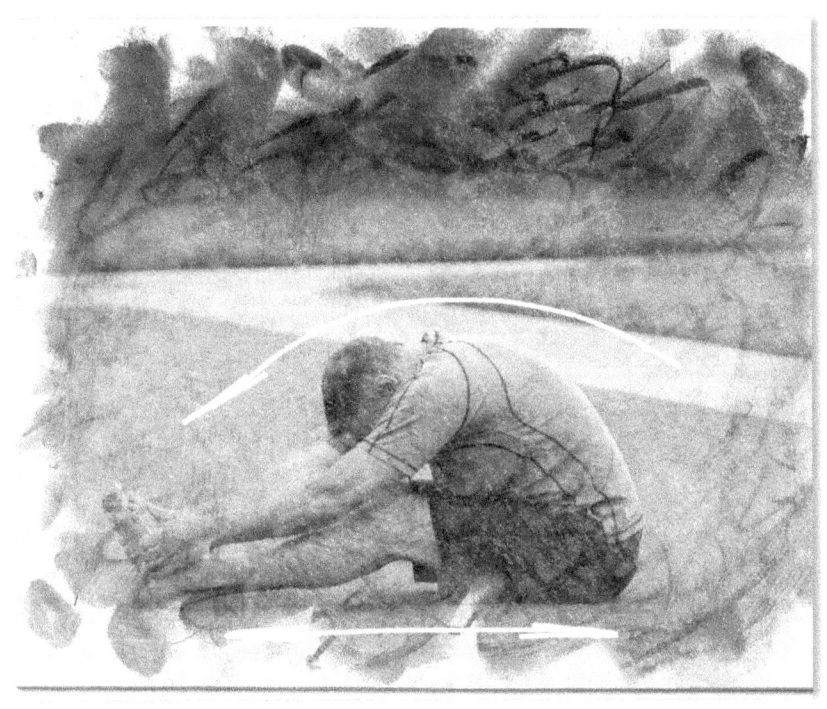

Fig 29
Legs and back, head down, stretch the torso.

Here, one of the most important focusing points is the shoulder blade, which is worked as the foot tied to the ipsilateral hand is pointed, pulling and stretching the shoulder and the shoulder blade area. This is one of the very few times one unrelated region is used to stretch against another, as most exercises have agonist stretch the antagonist.

1. In a sitting position, grab hold of your feet.

2. Straighten your legs out.

3. Take a DDB, hold the air for 15 seconds as you bring your head closer and closer to the ground, and then for additional 10 seconds, attempt to bring the head even closer to the ground.

Here you are also focusing not just on the legs, but also the neck and the back.

With the head hanging towards the ground, allow the gravity to pull as you focus on stretching the fascia on the posterior of your neck and upper back. Here the pointing of the feet in alternating fashion may also work the shoulder blades.

There is a tiny little shoulder blade muscle some call the infraspinatus, located on the bottom and posterior part of the shoulder blade. This area is very difficult to stretch and plays a big role in tight fascia, contributing to many neck and shoulder problems. You can work them quite effectively performing this exercise one leg at a time even on a couch while watching a show.

Repeat this exercise as needed to release tension in shoulders and upper back, low back, and legs.

22. The Great Glute Release

If mind is in charge, then who is in charge of the mind?
Better yet, what is the mind?

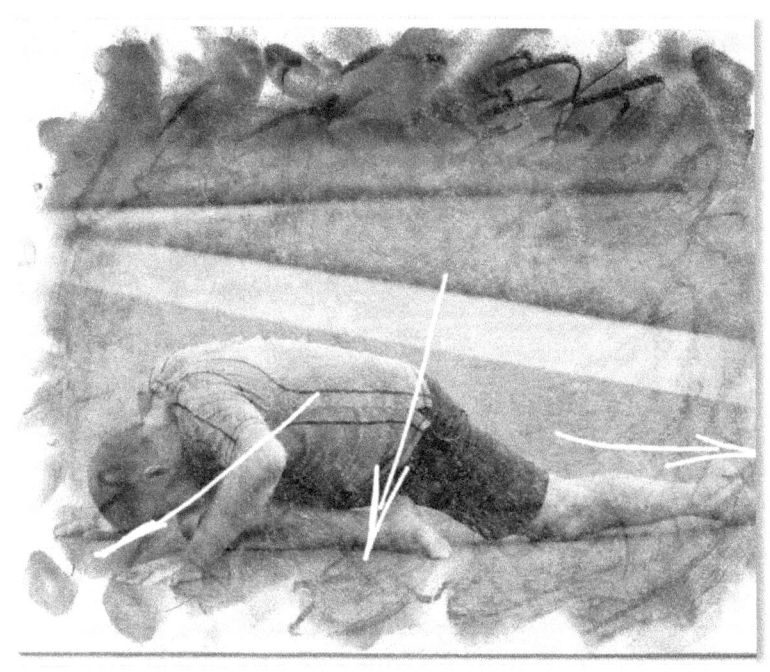

Fig 30

The great glute release

This is one of the most if not the most important maneuvers in releasing the fascia in charge of back issues. I recall one of patients in my early years of my practice. He had a 12-millimeter disc bulge at his L5. The disc itself and the bones right above and below could not be touched due to sensitivity and danger of damage to the very important life data carrying nerve root being compressed by the disc. I recall adjusting his mid-back and doing this stretch for him. It took us a couple of months, but the next MRI showed a 10-millimeter correction now down to 2 millimeters. This exercise, I'm convinced, altered DL's ability to walk and perform. He was able to get married and live happily ever after.

1. Fold one leg under torso.
2. The other leg is posteriorly stretched.
3. Put pressure on butt with leg folded.
4. DDB 15/10

23. Leg Up On Stabilizing Core

Can you imagine beyond that which you already know and create a new thought?

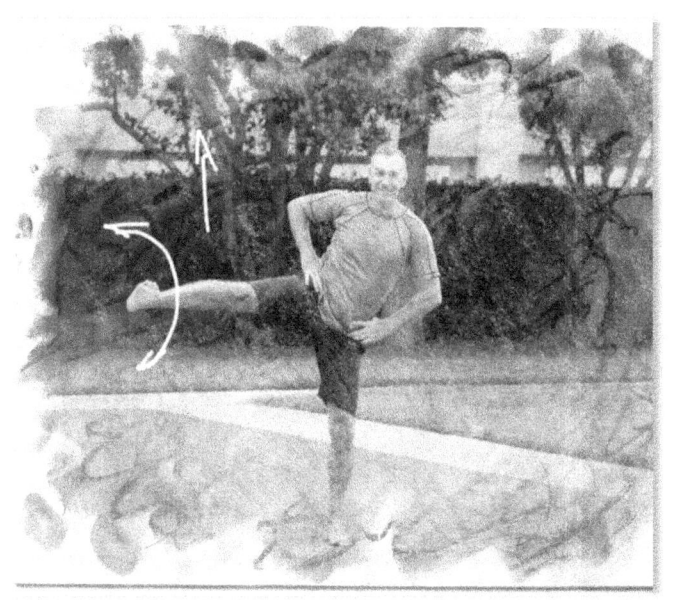

Fig 32a

You can raise your leg from side and back. Bilaterally, using DDB 15/10 system, this exercise is an offshoot of the imaginary wall exercise. It fires up muscles hardly used.

1. Raise the leg sideways to its limit.

2. Bring your toes back and stick your heel out

3. DDB and for 15/10, continue to elevate, to your ability.

4. Repeat with internal and external rotation of foot.

5. Proceed to elevate and repeat steps above in front and back. Feel free to experiment in 45-degree angles as well. This will fire up muscles you may have not used for years, if ever, increase tone, and strengthen your core.

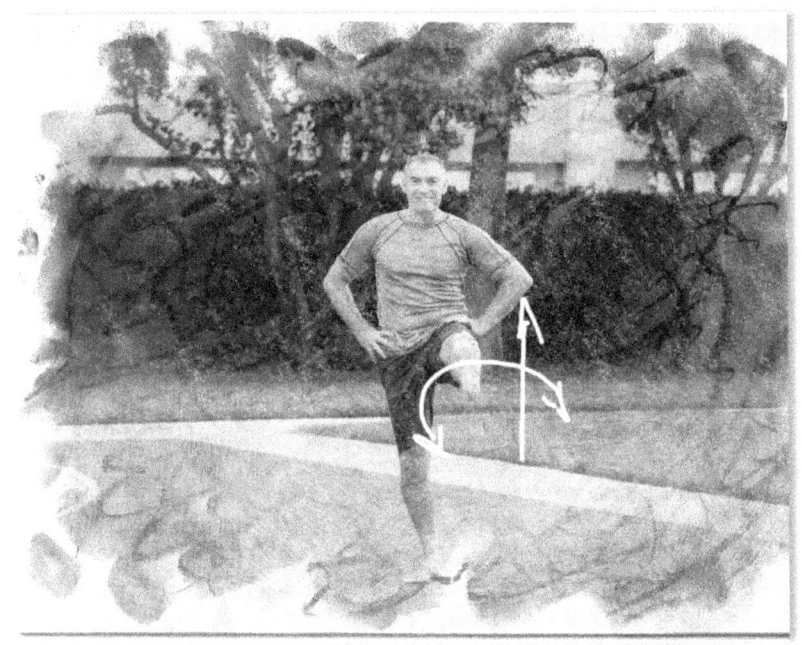

Fig 32 b

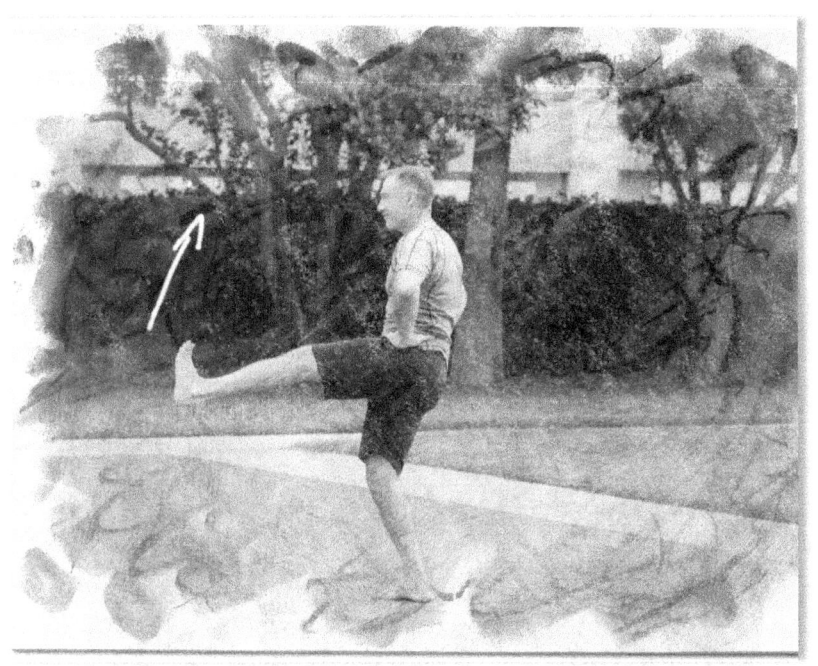

Fig 32 c

Posterior Leg Up is of great benefit and may be performed in couple of ways.

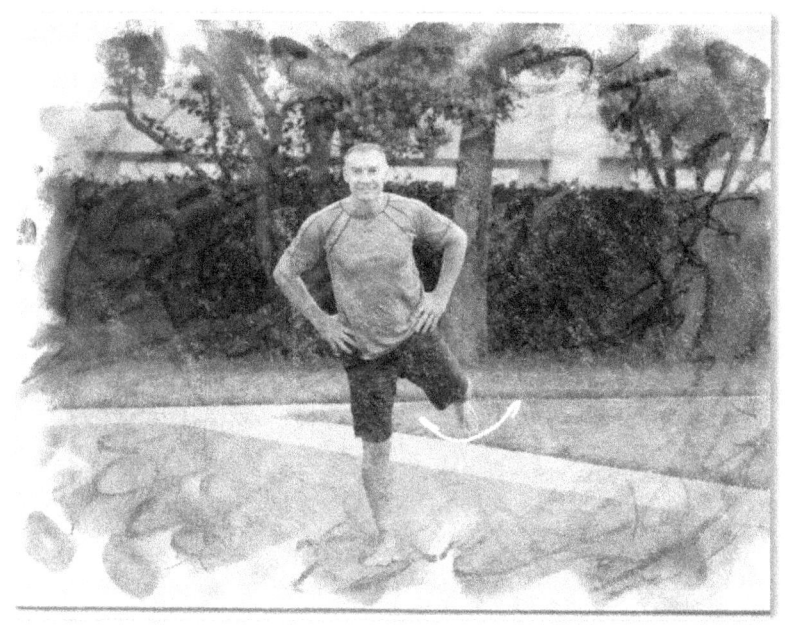

Fig 33 a

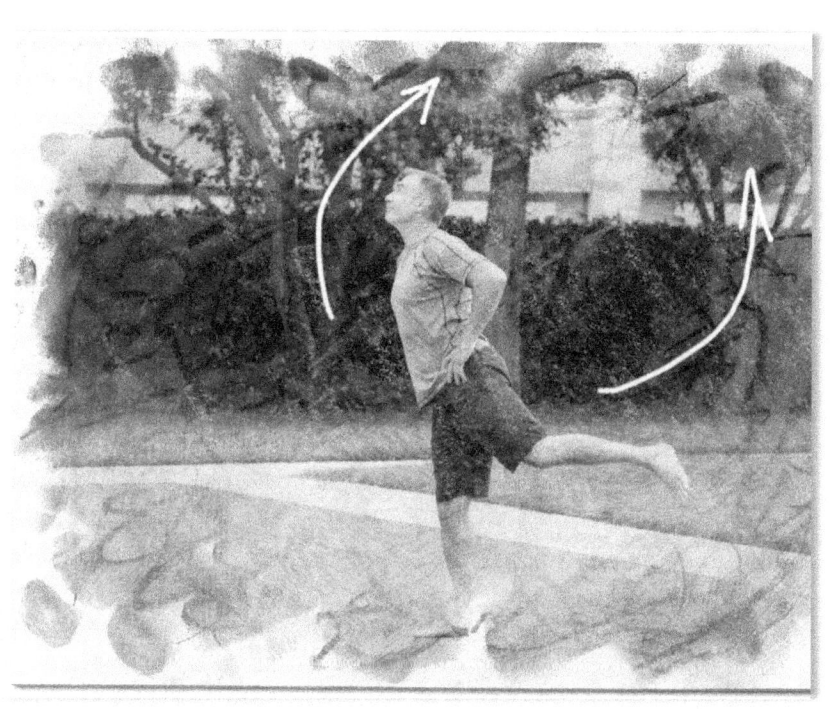

Fig 33 b

1. Elevate the legs, back up towards the wall, then focus on taking your foot towards the sky, one at a time to keep from falling, to highest point.

2. Use DDB with 15/10 system. Posterior leg raise to maximum, DDB for 15 seconds.

3. Bend backwards to approximate head to the heel.

4. Repeat with external and internal rotation of the foot for maximum results.

5. Repeat as often as needed to strengthen core.

6. As a variant, grab ankle to support and balance, but don't approximate foot to body; instead, push foot towards the sky.

Epilogue

Practiced properly, doing DDB 15/10 with intended intensity can serve as a total workout. It can enhance performance for boxers, UFC fighters, military personnel, from an elite athlete to the older crowd attempting to stay young. It can mobilize your joints and restore your ability to move them. It can restore and enhance strength, oxygenate your entire body, and improve total health and flexibility. You can choose to do all of these as a total intense workout or choose a couple that work for you that may assist in a particular ailment. If you choose just one exercise and if that one changes your life for the better, I have accomplished my goal.

The whole game is played out in your mind, the energy of life, the feelings, the love, or the drama.

About the Author

Dr. Eric Pastrmac DC ND was an aerospace engineer that became a chiropractor and a board certified Doctor of Naturopathy. He is a member of the Bolivian Natural Medical Society Sobometra. Dr. Pastrmac DC ND melds his Senior Design Aerospace Engineering background with human spinal mechanics and understanding of soft tissue and fascia behavior to bring forth most effective healing self-help system, DDB 15/10.

www.ingramcontent.com/pod-product-compliance
Lightning Source LLC
Chambersburg PA
CBHW070355290526
45790CB00004B/1505